MW00895237

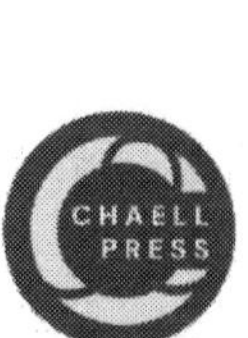
CHAELL
PRESS

CHARISE JEWELL

# Crazy

MEMOIR
OF A
MOM
GONE
MAD

Crazy: Memoir of a Mom Gone Mad / Charise Jewell
Edited by Shannon Moroney
Originally published by Dixi Books 2021
Chaell Press edition published 2024

ISBN 978-1-7383709-0-0 (paperback)
ISBN 978-1-7383709-1-7 (ebook)

chaellpress.com
charisejewell.com

Dedicated to E, A, J, and S.

# AUTHOR's NOTE

This book is based on my experiences, memories, observations, opinions, and perspective. During some of these events I was sleep-deprived, heavily medicated, and/or experiencing psychotic delusions. My recollections and interpretations may differ from those of others. I have confirmed facts as much as possible, using medical records and interviews. Names and personal details were changed to protect privacy. Some conversations have been shortened or abridged, however the meaning has been preserved. This is my story, the way I remember it, and from my point of view.

# CONTENTS

# PROLOGUE: The Feast

"Dinner's ready," I announce excitedly, to no one in particular. I look down into the pot as I call out, and this amplifies my voice, although it doesn't need it. I'm usually soft-spoken but over the past few days I've developed the ability to project loudly without even trying. It's only one of many newly discovered talents, like culinary skills that are all coming together from years of knowledge combined with previously hidden natural abilities. Out of the blue it seems that I have an instinctive ability to blend flavours and to time each step perfectly. The resulting meals could be served in gourmet restaurants. I don't usually cook on a Friday night, but this weekend is Mother's Day, and I'm in the mood to celebrate. I don't know exactly why I have so much energy and enthusiasm when I've hardly been sleeping lately, but I'm just going to enjoy it. Eric and the children always make Mother's Day special for me, so this dinner tonight is my way of pre-emptively expressing my gratitude. I've spent hours in the kitchen, tapping into my creativity and the joy of cooking. I can't wait to enjoy my family's praise.

I hear Suzie clamber up the stairs from the basement playroom with Alex close behind her. At ages four and ten, they have boundless energy but they don't always come right away when they're called. As they burst into the kitchen, my excitement grows. They're hungry, and they are in for a treat. This might be the best meal I've ever made.

"What's for dinner, Mommy?" they ask.

"It's a surprise!" I say with a big smile as I stir the pot one more time. It's full of bright colours, which please my eyes, but the aroma makes my nose think something is missing. It smells delicious, but there is something I could add to make it just that much better. One more thing to give it that extra oomph.

"Rosemary," I say to Suzie, snapping my fingers.

"What, Mommy?" she asks, eyebrows up and slight confusion in her voice.

"This dish needs rosemary," I say, grabbing a twig hanging from the stove's fan hood with one hand and the nearby kitchen scissors with the other. I start snipping away above the pot. "Good thing we dried this out earlier, hey Suze?"

She nods in agreement. My daughter loves doing just about anything with me, which I think is mainly because she's the youngest of three and the only girl. But I've been so focused on my writing and my art lately that I haven't had a lot of time to play with her, and when we do play I'm usually too irritable from lack of sleep. When I suggested that we dry out some of the herbs from our indoor garden this morning, her eyes lit up. She beamed with pride to be trusted with the "adult" scissors, captivated by how I attached each branch to the fan hood with only a magnet and a binder clip and explained the properties and flavours of each plant from our garden. Properties and flavours that I never realized I knew. She was in awe of me. I was in awe of myself.

My kids love it when I have new ideas—they're often amazed. Lately I've had endless ideas, so they've been in a constant state of amazement. Because of me. Because I'm amazing. I've never felt better. This will be my eleventh Mother's Day and I've finally got this motherhood thing down.

"I have a joke for you." I smile at the two little faces staring up at me with their big, curious eyes. "What do you get when you cross an INFJ engineer with a mom?"

They stare at me, confused. They have no idea what Myers-Briggs personality typing is. I don't give them time to guess before I blurt out the punchline.

"A logical, emotional, multi-tasking, hyper-efficient, superstar!"

My joke falls flat. Maybe I should explain the Myers-Briggs theory to them. They probably don't remember when I was a mechanical engineer because I haven't worked since we moved to Calgary for Eric's job. It might be too confusing. This suggests they're not ready to learn that I can sometimes predict the future.

Our neighbour's dog barks in their yard, snapping me out of my reverie and waking up my senses again. I'd been distracted by my lovely children, and the bark reminded me to be on alert. The universe is looking out for me. I glance around for signs of imminent danger as the smell of dinner permeates into my nostrils. It smells sublime. Wait—it smells done. Like one more minute and it will burn! What happened to the timer I set to tell me when everything is cooked? Did I forget to set it?

DING.

I heave a sigh of relief and satisfaction. Just when I think I couldn't be any more on my game the universe confirms that I've got this. Impressive.

"Can you guys set the table, please?" I ask. "And use the cloth napkins. I wonder where your brother is?" I turn the stove off, remove the pot from the burner, and dump its ingredients into the Crockpot in one smooth motion. The Crockpot contains a chicken, the meat, the protein, the highlight of the feast. I retrieve the ladle from its spot beside the stove and begin to blend everything together. The colours are stunning. The smell is perfect. It's going to be delicious.

"Jack!" I call loudly, just as he saunters into the kitchen. My eight year-old rarely hears me the first time, and is seldom interested in stopping whatever he's doing to come and eat.

"Yes?" He smiles with the thrill of having one-upped me. I ignore him, too focused on the tasks at hand.

"Oh, good, you're here. Can you get your milk, please?" I turn to Alex. "Alex, pour some for you and Suzie, please."

I'm talking quickly because I don't want to miss a beat as every moment leads to the climax: the presentation of my mouthwatering creation. The kids hustle to do as I've asked. They are as eager to please me as I am to please them.

"Eric, dinner!" I call my husband of fifteen years. He is going to be floored. I lift the ceramic pot out of its electric shell, carry it to the round, glass kitchen table, and place it down gently in the centre just as my boys return carrying drinks, Eric walks up from behind and gives me a quick hug, and Suzie finishes arranging the napkins and cutlery just-so. I lift off the lid dramatically and we watch the steam rise up. I insert the ladle into my fantastic stew and begin to scoop serving after serving into each person's bowl. I am so hungry and eager for this celebration with my darlings.

At first, no one says anything, and I take this as the highest praise. They are speechless! I feel myself beaming with pride. Eric is the first to speak.

"What's this?" He stares down at his bowl in disbelief. Then he looks up at me and it's hard to read his expression. I can't tell if he is bewildered or bemused, but neither is the reaction I expected. I look around at the rest of my adoring family. Jack looks flummoxed, Suzie looks disgusted, and Alex looks almost scared. I feel something in my heart clench as I realize that they are not impressed. I've been working for hours and they're still not impressed.

"What do you mean?" I ask, my voice sounding shrill and defensive even to my own ears. "It's dinner. It's the dinner I've been cooking all afternoon. Doesn't it smell terrific?" Alex picks up his spoon and gingerly moves my concoction around in his bowl, but he doesn't raise it to his mouth. I look down at my own serving, see the rainbow of colours and breathe in the tantalizing smell. I, for one, am salivating. I'm ready to dive in, but then I notice the bones. Why didn't I see the bones when I scooped it into my bowl? I look back to the Crockpot. Why is there a chicken carcass but no meat?

"Dinner?" Eric finally says. "I don't think so." He shakes his head. I'd lost all track of time over the last few hours—the last few days, really—minutes and hours rushing past in a blur. Now time grinds to a halt. What is he talking about? Of course it's dinner. What else would it be? Why is he criticizing me in front of the children like this? We can just take the bones out. Leaving them in is an honest mistake. I probably didn't want to waste the marrow.

"Just put the bones on the side and eat it," I instruct, trying to make light of my mistake. I reach for my spoon and dig deep to scoop up my first bite, but what I lift out of the bowl surprises me. It's a small piece of an orange peel. A blood orange peel. I don't remember adding that. I'm taken aback, but I don't let it show. I can't let them doubt me. I can't doubt myself. It must have been stuck to the cutting board. It could happen to anyone. Lately everything has been going so well. For the past week or so everything I've touched has turned to gold. This is nothing to read into.

"Guys, just eat." I insist. I lift my spoon to my mouth and Alex follows suit, both of us tasting at the same time while everyone else continues to stare, dumbfounded. He nibbles at the last remaining bit of meat on a bone. My orange peel tastes awful—bitter, rotten, and tough—but I force myself to chew and swallow, pretending nothing's wrong.

"Don't eat it, Alex." Eric reaches to take the bone away from him. "Nobody eat anything. This is garbage."

I can't believe he would insult me this way, especially with everybody watching. In the eighteen years we've known each other my husband has never publicly humiliated me. My entire body starts to tense up, my hands begin to tremble, and my cheeks flush. I look down into my bowl while I try to figure out what to do, and that's when I see it. That's when I see that he is right. It is garbage, literally. Chicken bones, carrot peelings, strawberry tops, apple cores, pepper stems and seeds, corn silk, orange peels, kiwi skin, and tea bags. All sprinkled with rosemary. My head starts to spin.

I scramble to recover the moment—the moment I've been anticipating all day. My perfect Mother's Day weekend dinner. *Recover this, Charise, recover.* Panic rises. *Think!*

"Gotcha!" I stand up. "It was a joke!" My cheeks turn even more red. My hands shake. I fold them together so no one will notice. I wait for everyone to laugh, but they don't.

"Take your bowls to the counter, kids," Eric says calmly. "I'll order pizza."

Everybody stands and starts to bustle around the kitchen and it's all just too busy for me. There is too much noise. I retreat to the dark, quiet dining room and sit in the vintage lounge chair I inherited from my grandparents. I need comfort. I look at the evergreen tree out the window, catatonic. I hear a muffled conversation between Eric and the kids, then him on the phone placing an order for pizza. How did this happen? How did my brilliant mind let this happen? I have to figure it out. Was my overtired mind simply suffering from lack of sleep? How could I be hitting it out of the park with everything else and suddenly have this colossal failure? What kind of woman makes her family dinner out of compost? How did I not realize that I was cooking garbage as I took it from our compost bin? Have I gone crazy?

# PART ONE: *Mania*

*May 2017*

# 1. Decadent Desserts

"Why is Daddy taking so long in the bathroom?" Suzie asks. I pull my gaze away from the stained glass windows, cheap chandeliers, and intimidatingly large clock hanging near our table, to make eye contact with Suzie, who is absentmindedly eating her dessert. The kids seem to have forgotten about last night's dinner fiasco, and eating here at The Old Spaghetti Factory in downtown Edmonton has been a perfect antidote. This morning Eric had questioned whether we should still travel for his hockey tournament or if it was better for us to stay home so I could rest. I insisted we go, and pointed out laughingly: We're Canadian. We don't miss hockey. It had been the right decision so far. The kids read or played on their iPads during the three hour drive, and then we'd checked into the Fantasyland Hotel inside the giant West Edmonton Mall. A mini break is just what we all need right now.

"What?" I ask.

"Why is Daddy taking so long?" Suzie repeats.

"He's not in the bathroom, sweetie. He's going to meet us back at the room."

"Why?"

"He went for a massage in the mall, remember?"

Realization creeps across Suzie's face and she nods her head thoughtfully before returning her attention to her bowl of ice cream. It's finished, but she scrapes the spoon across the bottom to pick up any remaining liquid. Jack's barely touched his dessert. He sits beside me, mesmerized by the clock on the wall.

"Can we go?" Alex asks, pushing his bowl away. It still has ice cream in it. I point and give him a quizzical look before taking another sip of wine.

"I'm too full."

I smile and reach for his leftovers, happy to finish my meal with something sweet. But the first bite doesn't taste right on my tongue, which is strange because I always love dessert. I raise my glass to my mouth but as I inhale the bitter twang I realize that I don't want anything more to eat or drink. I'm struck by the feeling of satiation in a way that I've never been before in my life. I don't want to drink the rest of my wine, but I don't want it to go to waste.

"Do you guys want to do an experiment?"

Three sets of eyes meet mine, intrigued.

"What kind of experiment?" Alex asks, skeptical because he knows enough about science to know that experiments require work.

"What do you think it would taste like to mix ice cream and wine?"

They stare at me, then at the dishes in front of me, eyes wide open and smiles playing on their mouths. Alex says gross, Jack tells me to try it, and Suzie seems too stunned to say anything. She's used to me insisting on proper behaviour, especially in a restaurant. I drop the rest of the ice cream into the wine with an unceremonious plop. It doesn't fizz or bubble or do anything remotely exciting. It's rather anticlimactic. I stir it with the only clean knife on the table, and then take a sip.

"What does it taste like?"

I swish the liquid around in my mouth before swallowing.

"Not good. Want to try?"

Alex and Suzie refuse, but Jack wants a taste.

"Sorry, Jack, I meant Alex. You're too young."

"So's he!" Sulking. And he's right.

"Think we can do anything else to make it taste better?" I ask.

They offer up the last morsels from the table. Jack's vanilla ice cream. Eric's abandoned beer, two French fries. I mix and taste after each addition, to the shocked and delighted eyes of my children. We all laugh loudly now. I love being Fun Mommy. I declare the concoction Officially Disgusting, and Jack and I try to persuade Alex to try one little sip. He refuses, no matter how many times we ask. I feel slightly disappointed that he is so averse to taking a chance, but I'm also proud. I hope he will be equally adamant when his friends eventually try to pressure him into trying drugs and alcohol.

Eric already paid the bill, so we get ready to leave. An older man at the table behind us stares at me as I turn to reach for my sweater—his look is one of sobering judgement and displeasure. I try to ignore him, but the smile falls off my face.

It's only once we're back out in the mall that I realize I've left behind the napkin art I'd doodled while we'd waited for our meal. Alex offers to run back for it, so the rest of us return to wait on the bench in the foyer. My head still spins from the neighbouring diner's disapproving glance. The only eye contact I've had from other men lately is lustful and wanting. In addition to all my newfound talents, my sensuality is in full bloom. I've never felt more attractive in my life. It upsets me that this man's eyes were so disapproving, rattles me like last night's compost stew. I reach into my purse for my phone to call Eric, but it isn't there.

"I found it!" Alex holds up the napkin with my drawing of a dying tree. Maybe that was the problem. Maybe drawing sinister things calls forth sinister forces.

"Awesome! Thanks Alex!"

I remain seated, still rummaging for my phone, when a sinking feeling hits. I'd left my purse unzipped on the bench throughout dinner. I'd noticed that it was open but lately the universe has been protecting me, because I am good, so I decided not to close it. A group of teenagers ate at the table beside us, one of them sitting near my purse. It would have been easy for him to reach into it without my noticing, especially during our ice cream experiment.

"So, can we go?" Alex asks, staring at me.

"I think I lost my phone. Can you please go and check around the floor and bench near where we were sitting?"

He runs off, happy to be given another task, and I stand up to go and speak to the hostess. It feels like something a responsible person would do. When she's finished taking down Eric's number in case it's turned in, I head back to our table with Jack and Suzie. Alex is still searching. The man is still there. He is still staring. Still judging.

"Any luck?" I ask while leaning down to look.

"No, I can't find it."

Alex stands. There is nothing left for us to do but leave.

"Oh well. It's just a phone. At least you found my art!" I say this loudly for the evil man to overhear, because I'm starting to like the idea of his disapproval and want to encourage it, but I also mean it. My phone can be replaced, but I don't want this negativity to replace the fun memories we just made. We walk out. I hold my head high.

## 2. Risky Behaviour

Eric found my phone back in our hotel room. It was easy to find—he just dialed my number. I must have left it behind when we went for dinner. I left it again when we put the kids to bed and went for a walk, because Eric has his phone and I have Eric. He is my hero. We closed the door behind us and headed out for some quality adult time. The kids are happy for parent-free time. This mall is too crowded and part of me wishes I were back upstairs with them, avoiding all this chaos. I don't remember much of West Edmonton Mall from when we visited eight years ago, although that was during the day when there were more children enjoying the rides. Now it's mostly teenagers and adults, all of them looking for their version of a good time. The hot-air balloon Ferris wheel looks familiar, and the roller coaster, but I don't remember it being so loud. Everyone is pushing, trying to get somewhere, trying to get something. Eric walks slightly ahead of me and clears a path for us. If I didn't feel his hand holding mine I'd get lost. Or tempted away.

I'm wearing my new shirt, the one I bought a few hours ago with Jack and Suzie on our way back to the room after dinner, and every person who walks past me notices. It's a short-sleeved slightly see-through yellow peasant blouse that looked innocent on the hanger, before I paired it with a black bra and slipped the sleeves down to bare my shoulders. I don't normally dress provocatively but lately something keeps telling me to be more bold, to take more chances, and it feels good. I've always enjoyed sex and being sexy, but for some reason I no longer feel the need to downplay it like I usually do. I want to embrace it. Clearly, the men around me appreciate my efforts—even the young ones walking through the mall with their girlfriends turn to do a double-take. They don't care that I'm a forty year-old mother of three.

Eric makes a sharp right turn and we veer into a shoe store. I breathe deeply, relieved to step out of the noise and attention. I like turning heads but it gets tiresome.

"What are we doing?" I ask. "Do you need new shoes?"

"You said you saw some that you liked."

"I did?" I have no recollection of a conversation about shoes. Eric nods.

"You said that while you were walking back to the room you noticed some sexy shoes in one of the store windows."

I furrow my eyebrows and try to remember making this statement. Nothing. I shrug my bare shoulders.

"Okay, well, we're here. Let's look at shoes." Eric points to a shelf nearby. "Do you like those?" He's pointing at a pair of Steve Madden open-toe mules with four inch heels. Perforated tan leather wraps the top of the foot but lets the toes and circular cut-outs of skin peek through. My daughter and I talk about being fierce, which I've described to her as a combination of tough and beautiful. These shoes are sexy fierce, and they're nothing I would normally buy, but right now they look more alluring than anything else in the store. I try them on and the cuffs feel like shackles, which I like. Lately I've been wondering if I was a dragon in a former life, and the familiarity of these shoes makes me think that I was. With both approval and desire in his eyes, Eric watches me catwalk up and down the aisle. I can't wait to wear them out of the store. I have never worn heels this high.

Eric decides to browse, and I eagerly accept the challenge to find him something equally sexy. I never noticed how sexy men's shoes were before tonight.

"What about these ones? I like the blue laces."

"I need brown shoes."

"They are brown shoes."

"The laces are too much."

I don't think they're too much. I think they're hot as hell and if he wore them with one of his suits he'd turn just as many heads as I do. But I don't want to argue. He is stubborn, my husband, and over the years I've learned that if it doesn't really matter then it's not worth trying to persuade him. I sit down and he takes his sweet time until he finally finds the right pair. Then he pays for our shoes, and the salesgirls flatter us with compliments. It's almost closing time and if I were them I would hustle us along, but Eric eats it up, lingering and laughing.

"What's so funny?" I ask, looking from a salesperson, who is giggling like a schoolgirl, to Eric, who is chuckling like an idiot, and back. I must have missed the joke. I stare at her curiously, with neither jealousy or malice, because there is simply nothing for me to be jealous of. She is chubby and plain, with dumpy clothes, and a pig-snout shaped nose. Her eyes are beady and sunken, her skin has old acne scars, and her limp brown hair needs highlights and layers. She has no style, no sustenance. Her name tag is hidden by her lacklustre locks, but I'm sure it would be perfectly unremarkable like everything else about her. I search Eric's face for a clue as to why he's playing along, but there is none. He would respond to anyone who flatters him, no matter how underwhelming or unattractive she is. I roll my eyes and shake my head before walking away, towards the front of the store. Let him have his kicks.

The air in the shoe store has changed and I feel stifled. There's also a growing stench of some kind. I walk back into the mall and immediately notice that the crowd has thinned out. Most of the stores are closed. All of the nearby posters advertise sex, plain and simple. Of course it's more complicated, because the scantily-clad pre-pubescent models pretend to advertise clothes, makeup or jewelry, but I see through it. I feel tired, but I don't want to go back to our room just yet. I lean against the glass storefront and look down to admire my new shoes and alluring red toenails.

"Ready to go?" Eric asks, emerging from the store and propping his elbow out for me to take hold of. It's a good thing he's here, the men walking past were already starting to ogle me. Starting to wonder if I was alone or if they should approach. That could have been fun. But I've had enough fun for the night. I just want to enjoy my husband without all this filth and smut making everything dirty. I just want wholesome love right now.

"Yes. Where to?"

"Follow me," he smiles through a playfully commanding tone. I link my arm through his and we start to strut. Life is good.

With the stores closing, we head to Eric's truck to continue our date since the kids are in the hotel room. Alex has my phone and will call us if there's a problem. All three children are either asleep or enjoying extra TV right now. Everyone loves it when Eric and I have a date.

He holds my door open, like a gentleman, and I kiss him on the cheek before climbing in. I kick my new shoes onto the floor mat and recline my chair. Eric walks around the front, climbs into the truck, rolls down the windows, opens the glove compartment, and pulls out a vape pen. I forgot that a month ago we had a conversation about trying one, just for fun. Just to break out of our suburban parent stereotype for a moment. I feel too drunk to contribute anything to the figuring out of this new device, which is strange because I haven't had anything to drink since dinner, now hours ago. Maybe I'm just tired. Over the past two weeks, I've been sleeping less and less, to the point where a four hour stretch feels refreshing. Last night I managed three hours.

"Did you get it?" I say. I'm growing impatient.

"Yeah, here you go." He passes it to me and explains how to use it using too many words. My brain currently cannot absorb anything he's saying, so I fiddle with the button until something happens and I inhale. The taste is weird and I don't know what to do since it doesn't feel like a cigarette, which is what we usually smoke to be badasses. Do I hold it? Exhale? Soon enough I have to breathe so I release the fumes, which also smell weird, and pass it back to Eric. I don't feel anything. We trade it back and forth and it starts to feel slightly more natural, but I still don't feel much. I wish we'd stuck to cigarettes.

"We should stop," Eric says as he stares at the liquid level through the glass.

"Okay." I shrug. I watch him put everything away and then roll up the windows.

"What do you want to do now?" I ask. I know we have to get back to the kids but I want to savour this moment. And I know they're fine. Normally after a cigarette I just want to sit, enjoy the buzz coursing through my body, and watch whatever images appear behind my closed eyes. But tonight, I feel antsy. I'm not ready for the night to end. I don't want to lie in bed listening to everyone sleep while I struggle with insomnia. I lift one leg up onto the dashboard and turn to face Eric while I subtly pull down the sleeves and neckline of my blouse.

"You know, I had a lot of fun back there the other day." I nod my head towards his truck's backseat.

"You did, did you?" Eric turns to look at me, smiling coyly, resting his head back against his headrest.

"It seemed like you had a lot of fun too if I remember correctly." I give him my best wanton look. It never fails. I think part of the reason men like it so much is because I come across so innocent. I'm small, brunette, and fresh-faced—the girl next door. They are pleasantly delighted by my sexual desire and expertise. Men are often surprised to discover that women love sex just as much as they do.

"I did indeed have fun." Eric's eyes twinkle.

Just the thought of our recent backseat romp is enough to rile me up again. A few days ago, back in Calgary, we went for a couples' massage, and the masseuse touched me so firmly yet so tenderly that I almost had an orgasm just by her rubbing my shoulders. As we drove home, I told Eric. He parked in our garage, and we barely got our seatbelts off before climbing on top of each other and over the armrest into the back seat. It was incredible.

"So?" I raise my eyebrows and smile provocatively.

Eric looks around nervously.

"We're in a public parking garage!" He is obviously just as eager as I am to rip off our clothes, but also obviously more level-headed.

I shrug. He just needs some convincing.

"What if someone walks by?"

"You have tinted windows." I make a show of starting to caress my neckline, lingering slowly at the middle. So cheesy, but it always works, even when I do it as a joke. His eyes follow my fingertips and he starts to breathe hard.

"There's a light right there." He points out the front window, still not lifting his eyes from my cleavage.

"No one will see. No one will even pass by." My voice is tender, soft, and I reach for him as I start to lift one foot over the armrest. He takes my hand and starts to follow me, but then stops and sits down again.

"There are people in the car next to us." He faces forward and says it robotically, as though they can hear. As though he's been caught with a prostitute instead of his wife.

Motherfucker. I had him. I sit down hard on the armrest, which is almost satisfying given how much I want sex right now.

"Let's go back to the room," he whispers, pulling me into the front seat.

"The kids are in the room." I say flatly. There goes our night.

"They'll be asleep. We can go in the shower."

Magic words. My heart starts to race. Maybe I'll even wear this new blouse in the shower and after it's turned see-through and he's had enough of seeing through it, he can rip it off me and we can make love and fuck and do all of the things.

"That's a really good idea," I say, reaching for my shoes. I put them on and fly out of the truck so fast that he has to keep up. And he does. He wants me almost as much as every other man I see. Maybe even more.

# 3. Demons and Omens

"Okay, everyone, I need you to listen to me."

It's almost eight o'clock on Mother's Day, two days after our garbage dinner and the morning after a long, wild night. I spent most of it in the hotel room bed wide awake, lonely, and afraid of noises coming from the hall. The dark hours passed slowly as I listened to my family snore while watching the smoke detector LEDs blink. I noticed that the lights and shadows occasionally took on the eyes and shape of a dragon. The LEDs blinked in response to my yes or no questions, in green or red code. I needed answers. I asked about my recent conversion to Buddhism and belief in reincarnation. I asked if our loved ones were safe, as I have a strong feeling that somebody is in danger. I asked if I was pregnant, because my period is late, breasts feel tender, and I've been so euphoric. The dragon replied yes, yes, and definitely. My conversation with the lights kept me company, but I did have to wake Eric up a few times, for fun and out of fear. I told him stories from my childhood—secrets I'd never shared. I saw a ghost, which turned out to be the statue in the corner of our room that I'd decorated with hats and a bag, to mark our territory. Somebody in the hall jiggled our door handle and I was convinced they were trying to break in. Through it all, Eric was patient. He listened and comforted me as needed, and had sex on my command until he was too tired to respond. The less I slept, the more energy I had. My family finally woke up an hour ago and showered me with their Mother's Day gifts: crafts, flowers, and chocolate. I feel loved. I have to protect them. Only I know what's coming next. I've figured it out, and I need to take action but I don't want to alarm them.

"Don't be scared but we need to hurry. Something bad is going to happen. It could be here, in Fantasyland Hotel, or somewhere else in Edmonton, or on the road, I'm not sure." My voice sounds calm but urgent. "If we pack and leave quickly we'll be okay. We just have to stay together."

Four confused and concerned faces stare at me.

"What about the water park?" Alex says.

"I'm sorry but we can't. We have to leave."

Eric wordlessly starts to pack. He's been silent through the gifts and pampering. He looks frustrated, as though he's more disappointed than the kids that we'll miss the water park. And tired. Yeah, he looks tired. I'm probably tired too but I don't feel it. I feel alive. The morning sunshine brought peace and comfort after the long, lonely night. I'm excited too, certain I'm pregnant. My stomach churned all night and my period is far too late. I'm also sad, because I'm sure something bad happened in last night's darkness. Maybe to our parents or a sibling. Or our dog Piper, back in Calgary. Or maybe our house was broken into and burned to the ground. Either way, we have to get out of this city before something even worse happens. It's about to, I can tell.

"Okay, guys, let's pack." I adopt a tone of command. "Anything on the floor needs to be thrown away, it's bad."

I put on my Crocs before stepping off the bed because my feet aren't allowed to touch the floor either. It's one of the rules. I don't know where the rules came from but I'm lucky because I know what they are. Lucky and grateful.

"That's garbage," I tell Eric as he reaches for a pile of discarded clothes on the floor.

"It's just dirty. We don't have to throw things away just because they're dirty." His voice carries a patient yet annoyed tone. I watch apprehensively as he stuffs yesterday's soiled clothing into a plastic bag and puts the bag into the suitcase. My heart is pounding but nothing happens. Maybe Eric can bridge both worlds, the good and the bad, without consequences. He even touched the clothes with his bare hands and nothing happened. Maybe the plastic bag works as a shield. Maybe I have to pay more attention to material properties—natural versus synthetic—not just light versus dark and colour versus black and white. Materials can determine if something is good or bad. If plastic worked as a shield then it was good, even though it was synthetic. If white plastic is okay, is dark plastic? It can't be recycled. Maybe good is not always good and bad is not always bad. Maybe it's the balance. The yin and the yang. That's what I have to focus on.

Next I know, my family is standing at the door, ready to go, watching me. I'm ready too except for one thing: my Crocs. Definitely synthetic. And although the plastic bag helped us I'm unsure about my Crocs. They're navy blue and I wore them all weekend. They crossed over from yesterday's wholesome fun to last night's sinister pleasures. I can't take a chance. I carefully lean against the bed to put on socks and runners instead, making sure my bare feet never touch the floor. I kick the Crocs under the bed to be discovered by the cleaner in a few hours. Then we flee.

# 4. Garbage Art

An argument breaks out between Eric and me in the hotel's parking garage. He wants to eat breakfast and I want to go before our truck gets broken into. There are bad men lurking. Eric wins, but the kids and I pick at our food. As soon as we're finished I make everyone rush to the truck. The three-hour drive home starts to feel endless, so we stop at the Alberta Sports Hall of Fame to stretch our legs. It is peaceful, bright, and overwhelmingly calm. It feels like Church. It is exactly what I need. The kids are well-behaved. They grasp the gravity of the situation, like I do. We stop for gas and I decide to share the good news about my pregnancy with my family. They are more dazed than excited. I consider purchasing a pregnancy test en route, but I'm tired and I don't need to pay to confirm something I already know. They'll accept it soon enough. When we arrive home, I'm perplexed. Everything is just as it should be. There is no evidence of the chaos that I'd been anticipating.

The calm of the house makes me uneasy. It's a mismatch to my sixth sense. Eric and I phone our parents, but they have no bad news to report. No one is hurt, ill, or dead. Even our dog is okay. I feel exhausted. After lunch, the kids and Eric settle in on the family room couch to watch *Inside Out*. I retreat to our bedroom for a nap, but after lying down I no longer feel tired. I want to be with my family. I want to be safely surrounded by our circle of love, so I rise from the heavy duvet and walk back downstairs. I'm reluctant to join them on the couch, because I'm too restless to sit still, so I reach for the newspaper and sit at the kitchen table behind them. I turn to the crossword and glance at the clues, but my mind is too scattered to focus. I stand, pace, fetch a glass of water, look out the window, and then back to the newspaper on the table. Suddenly I know exactly what I want to do. I want to create. I grab the newspaper and flip through it, scanning each page quickly before turning to the next one. I rip out anything that looks appealing and discard the rest. Once finished, I bring my stack of pages to the wall between the kitchen and the family room, just behind the couch where my fabulous family sits, oblivious. The blank space on this wall has bothered me since we moved in. I rifle through the papers, crumpling and ripping and taping seemingly random articles onto the wall. I don't know what I'm creating—I'm just going on instinct—but a shape soon starts to emerge. I work my way up the wall, confident in my artistry. When I'm halfway through the pile of newspaper, it becomes obvious. It's a tree. I'm making a tree. With quiet but swift determination, I fashion branches out of wires and a bird from a binder clip. Some pieces fall to the floor, which inspires me to add a fire near the bottom with crumbled newspaper logs for seats.

The movie ends around the same time as my work is complete. I step back to admire my art, feeling a deep sense of satisfaction and pride.

Alex gets up from the couch and comes over to me, looking at my creation on the wall. "What's that?" he asks.

"You tell me." I smile.

The other children, sensing that something out of the ordinary is happening, join us. No one speaks.

"What does it look like to you?" I ask Suzie.

"I don't know," she says, shy delight apparent in her voice and on her face.

"To me it looks like an arrow," Alex says, his eyes searching mine for approval. I smile and nod, which makes him beam.

"I think it's a fire. A forest fire," Jack says with confidence.

"It could be," I say.

"Me too. I think it's a fire too," Suzie agrees.

"I can see that," Alex says. "But I still think it's an arrow."

We all stare at the wall.

"Do you want to know what I think it is?" I ask. There is a chorus of yesses.

"A tree."

They look from me to the wall and back, each child deep in thought. Eric is still on the couch. He hasn't said a word.

"When I made it I thought it was a tree. But now when I look at it I think it looks like an arrow and a fire, and also a tree. Isn't that interesting?" I'm an artist at my very own vernissage. "We all look at the same thing and see something different."

My little audience nods in agreement, happy to be treated like grown-ups.

"And who's to say who's wrong?" I ask. Art is subjective. Words are subjective. Labels are subjective. These big thoughts rush in and make my heart swell with pride for this tree, these children, this conversation. I created all of them. I feel so proud I might just burst.

## 5. The Spring Fairy

The sun paints the early morning Calgary sky with lustrous shades of pink and orange, unlike anything I'd seen back when we lived in Toronto. Night is almost over and since I don't sleep anymore I'm able to appreciate the sunrise while drinking my morning coffee, after I've put in at least an hour of intense, creative writing. The words appear in my mind faster than I can type them, and I can type fast. I've never been an early riser, but these days I jump out of bed with more energy than I've ever had in my life. It's funny because I struggle to fall asleep. I've been decluttering our house every night until late to tire myself out. I've been averaging three hours of sleep per night for the past two weeks. I'm a night owl and an early bird. It's exhilarating.

I decide to go out and feel the sunrise, so I grab our dog's leash to bring her with me on a walk. Piper used to have to make do with a quick pee in the backyard while I fed the kids and took them to school before I could take her for a long run. Now she gets a walk and a run. Life is good for our dog. And my children. And my husband. I am just killing it on all fronts, and everybody is reaping the rewards. I love life now that I don't have to waste time sleeping. Is this energy what people are talking about when they say life begins at forty? My birthday was only five months ago but so far this is the best decade yet.

It's a crisp May morning so I pull on a sweater before clipping on Piper's leash, and stepping outside.

"Good morning!" I say cheerfully to a couple strolling by on the sidewalk. They smile and stop to admire my dog before we continue on our way. There are many people already up and at 'em at what I used to think was an ungodly hour, and all of them are friendly and eager for a little small talk. The sun is so bright, sky is so blue, flowers are blooming, and birds are chirping. It looks and feels as though the entire world is glowing, especially the trembling aspen across the street, which is encircled by a resplendent golden aura. It looks like a halo. It catches my breath for a moment.

"Chirp, chirp, chirp!" I tweet to the birds as we continue to walk. There is a moment of silence before they chirp back. Suzie was the one who taught me how to talk to birds. My daughter is only four years old and she has taught me so much. So have my sons. Children are so much more intelligent than adults realize. I am so lucky to have three of them to teach me, each one with their own knowledge, talents, and intuition. And then there is Piper, my wonderful dog. I reach down to pat her head.

"Time to circle back," I say. She gives me a look of understanding, and we turn to head home. I don't know how long we've been gone—I do everything on gut instinct now, which seems in tune with Piper. Along with everything else impressive lately, we are completely in sync. Our language is made up of pats, pauses, clicks, and the tone of my voice. Paying attention and actually listening to each other has really helped both of us.

The side door swings open just as we arrive home. Eric smiles when he sees me coming up the walkway. An apprehensive smile.

"Oh, hi," I say.

"Where were you?"

"Walking Piper." I cross over the threshold and he steps aside to let me pass. He takes Piper's leash from me while I slip off my Birkenstocks and walk into the kitchen to wash my hands. The house feels stuffy. It's still asleep.

"You're up early," he says.

"I know. I had to write." I smile as I walk past him towards the kitchen table. Ever since announcing my intentions to pursue writing professionally a few months ago, life has felt more exciting. Ironically, I recently interviewed for an engineering job, just as I decided to stop pursuing engineering jobs. The universe is funny. I nailed the interview, even though I've given up on engineering. Come to think of it, they should be calling me any day now to offer me the job.

"How was your sleep?" Eric asks.

"Short," I say. "I couldn't fall asleep again so I unpacked more of the boxes in the basement that we've never gotten to." Two floors down from my sleeping family, so I don't have to worry about waking anyone up. I spend hours there every night. I put my music on shuffle and take my time. It's fascinating how my phone comes up with exactly the right playlist these days—that never happens. I feel just as in sync with my phone as I do with my dog. Whenever it gets glitchy or the battery is low, it reminds me to take a break because maybe I'm the one who's glitchy. Smart phone. Smart me for learning how to communicate with animals and technology, and making everything more effective and efficient.

"I found treasure last night," I say, gesturing towards the jewelry boxes on the table.

"You set the table?"

I nod. I forgot that I did that late last night before finally crashing to sleep. We don't set the table for breakfast. Oatmeal doesn't need fancy cutlery.

"Looks nice." Eric gives me a glance that I can't read. He is either saying that the table looks nice as a compliment, or because he's concerned. Based on everything that happened over the weekend in Edmonton, my guess is concern. Or fear. I can't expect him to understand the new me right away.

"Morning, Mommy," Jack says. He walks over to me. I wrap my arms around him and we share a tender hug.

"Hi sweetie-pie! I didn't hear you come down." I keep my hands on his shoulders, not ready to let go of my affectionate eight year-old.

"Is breakfast ready?" Jack asks. This simple question breaks the spell.

"Yes—can you please get Alex and Suzie? There's a surprise this morning!"

His eyes widen as his mouth forms a smile.

"A surprise?"

I nod. Eric watches both of us from where he stands beside the counter.

"What is it?"

"I can't tell you until all three of you are here."

"Okay, Mommy."

He hurries away, runs up the stairs, and excitedly calls for his brother and sister to get out of bed. They are not early birds like Jack and Eric and, apparently, me, so it takes him a while to rouse them from their cozy beds. But eventually he does and our little trio returns to the kitchen, rubbing their eyes.

"Guys! Guess what! The Spring Fairy came while we were sleeping!"

They look at me wearing expressions that clearly say, "What the hell are you talking about?" No one in this house has ever heard of the Spring Fairy. She is a figment of my imagination, created intentionally to inspire and delight my children.

"What's the Spring Fairy?" Suzie asks. "Is it like the Tooth Fairy?"

"Yes! They're cousins! The Spring Fairy comes when spring has finally arrived and brings gifts for all of the children in the house to thank them for their patience through winter."

Alex, still mostly asleep, stares at me with a furrowed brow. He knows there's no tooth fairy and he's clearly not buying it. But he also knows a gift is a gift no matter who it comes from, and he wants in.

"What kind of gifts?" Jack asks.

"Sit down and let's find out."

Up until now it seems that nobody has noticed the boxes resting on the table, including Eric, even though I specifically showed him.

Within seconds, each one of my beloved children is seated and has opened their treasure. Suzie holds up a crystal teardrop necklace. Her eyes are huge. Jack and Alex each pull out similar gold bracelets and both boys look from me to the bracelets to Eric.

"Wow," I say with a grin. It's so good to see the jewelry unpacked after two years. I can't even remember where it originally came from.

"Can we, like, wear this?" Suzie asks, her voice incredulous.

"No," I say with a sympathetic smile. The Spring Fairy should have thought of this complication. They are too valuable for the kids to lose.

"So, what do we do with it?" Alex asks.

Eric delivers each of our bowls of oatmeal. The cinnamon and blueberries smell so good, so fresh, and I am ravenous.

"Okay, guys, put them away so we can eat," Eric says. The kids look to me, desperation in their eyes.

"We'll figure out what to do," I say. "Just put them away for now and we can talk about it after school."

They comply as they usually do, and we have a nice, cheer-filled meal. I'm the first to finish and as I carry my bowl to the sink I try to remember what I'm supposed to do next. My new routine is so productive but sometimes confusing. My old routine, the one with more sleep and less efficiency, is a lot more familiar.

"I think I'll go have a shower," I say to Eric. This sounds like the right thing to do although I'm not entirely convinced. Don't I shower at night?

"Good idea," he says. "I'm going to work from home today. I'll take the kids to school."

Right. I usually get the kids to school. But there's something more, something else that it feels like I'm forgetting. Eric never works from home.

"Okay, but don't go without me," I say, starting to feel a flutter of nerves. "I want to take them to school too." This is true but it also feels worrisome. What am I missing? If I don't take them to school, what will happen? Come to think of it, if I have a shower, what will happen? They'll be down here in the kitchen, one big happy family, and I'll be upstairs in the shower, alone. Anything could happen. I could cut myself shaving. Or slip on those dumb slippery tiles, or the soap, and hit my head. I could pass out and no one down here would know. I could die! What if I accidentally on purpose cut myself shaving? I know it's a bad idea, but I could be powerless to stop it, because I just want to watch the blood mix with the water and the soap bubbles, to see if it's bright or dark, and to watch the patterns form. What if something else happens and I don't even know what it could be, but I die? They'll still be one big happy family, managing perfectly fine without me, just like they are right now. I don't want to be forgotten. I can't let them realize they don't need me anymore.

"Are any of you ready to come up and get dressed?" I say from the stairs, pretending to be calm.

"Not yet," Eric says after a moment. I turn my head to look at them, sitting together, eating and laughing. It's like I'm already gone—already dead—and they don't even care.

"Okay," I say softly. I look up the stairs, which are dark and menacing.

"I don't think I have time for a shower," I say. "I'll just get dressed and be right back."

"Okay," Eric says.

"If I'm not back in a few minutes, can somebody please come and check on me?"

To this, Eric turns his head. He sees me resting on the bannister for support, and gets up to walk down the hall towards me.

"Are you okay?" He puts both arms around me. I rest my head against his chest and inhale deeply, smelling him to feel good. And it works. Kind of. I feel like I can be upstairs by myself, at least to get dressed.

"I'm fine. Just tired."

"Okay. We'll come get you in a few minutes if you're not back."

I smile.

"Thanks."

He kisses me on the forehead before returning to the kitchen. I lift one foot up and place it on the first step, pause for a deep breath, and force myself to keep going. It gets easier. By the time I near the top, I run up the remaining stairs, because being downstairs is okay and I think being upstairs will be okay, but being *on* the stairs is not. It's purgatory. The possibility of that hits me hard. If these stairs are purgatory, then that would make upstairs heaven and downstairs hell. But my family is downstairs and they can't be in hell. Maybe the stairs are a bridge, and downstairs can be heaven just like south can be on top if we flip the map around, like Escher. Maybe we just need to defy gravity. Maybe we're defying gravity already.

I should have brought my tea up. Sometimes I think so hard that I feel pain in my frontal cortex. My brain literally hurts when I think too much. Bizarre. I wonder if that happened to Einstein or Socrates or any of the greats when they were about to have an "Aha!" moment. But I have to stop wondering. Even wondering hurts right now and it will only lead me down the path to thinking.

I open the closet, glance at my clothes, and pull out the first thing that looks appealing: a short-sleeved scarlet coloured pencil dress with white polka dots so miniscule that they are almost hidden. My mom sewed it for me when I was in university, and it makes me feel good. It makes me feel loved. Mother's day was yesterday, and it was her birthday as well, so the combination must be making me sentimental. Wearing this dress will feel almost like a hug from her, from three thousand kilometres away in Toronto. The only problem is the zipper is broken. It broke the last time I wore it, during a grief ceremony for the baby I miscarried twelve years ago, before Alex. Twelve years and twelve days ago to be precise. I'm not morbid, just good at remembering significant dates and doing quick math. It felt symbolic and appropriate to honour my mother and the little life that had been lost back then with this dress. It feels symbolic and appropriate today too.

I step into what is essentially now a piece of cloth with sleeves, and think about what to do. I consider that perhaps I shouldn't wear this dress today, perhaps I should properly fix the zipper first, but then decide to wrap a thin black belt around my waist to cinch the fabric together. Problem solved. I still have my pyjama pants on but I can't think of a satisfactory alternative and I feel too cold to remove them. I reach for my hair, quickly plaiting a flattering side braid (another talent I've just discovered) and then just as quickly, I apply a bit of make-up. I rarely wear make-up for school drop-off, but Eric's home today and I want him to think I look good.

And I do look good. I step back to admire my reflection and to decide on accessories. I put on my sterling silver necklace with engravings of my children's thumbprints, the one I had commissioned from a local jeweler when Suzie was a baby, my earrings with the children's birthstones, and the bracelet that my older sister gave me. She's a mom too, and I miss being close to her. With all this jewelry adorning me, I feel very connected to my family. I feel protected by the power of the amulets they have bestowed. The fact that my last name is Jewell is not lost on me. It's the most powerful symbol of all. I regard my sovereignty in the mirror. The only thing a little out of place are my pyjama pants. I'm not sure what to do about them.

"Time to go!" Eric calls from downstairs. His sharp tone means it's time to go now. Right now, this minute. There is no more time to think or prepare. The pants look strange with my fancy dress, but it doesn't matter. It's school drop-off. People go in pyjamas all the time. I grab my sweater, the one with long front segments that can hang or be wrapped to create different looks. I pull it on quickly and I glance at my reflection one last time. The sweater has draped itself perfectly—I look like I have wings, and the whole ensemble is perfection. I remind myself of a dragon. I look fantastic! I smile broadly. I am so proud, killing it on all fronts.

"Let's go!" Eric is losing patience.

"Coming!" I say as I hurry to the top of the stairs. I hold the banister railing and carefully take my time walking down each step. I don't want to slip and fall on the upside-down gravity-defying bridge, and the synthetic carpet makes it extra slippery.

"Ha-ha," I gloat, turning back towards the stairs after I step down onto the landing. It doesn't reply, or maybe it does but I'm no longer there to listen because I'm running towards the mudroom. My family is gone, but they've left the door open for me and I can hear them outside making their way to our detached garage, so I don't have to panic. I pull the door closed as I step onto the concrete slab porch outside. More steps to contend with on my quest to rejoin my family, and no railing to help, but there are only three and they are easier to navigate because they are wider and there's no stupid slippery carpet. I catch up to Eric, who turns and looks me up and down with an expression I've never seen but it must mean delight. Maybe we'll make love again after dropping the kids off. Spend time together. This is going to be a fun day!

## 6. Communication Breakdown

"I think I'll colour my hair," I say, "I want to go blonde." I chew my gum hard and blow the biggest bubble I've ever blown. It pops with a loud crack.

Eric glances at me while keeping both hands on the steering wheel. The look on his face suggests that my idea is preposterous. I guess he doesn't know that blondes have more fun.

"You should stop talking," he says. His voice sounds more defeated than angry.

"You should drive more carefully." I look out the window. "Where are we going anyway? Is it time to get the kids from school already?"

"We're going home. We took the kids to school and then went grocery shopping."

Oh, right. The friendly cashier kept laughing and telling Eric to buy me whatever I wanted when I kept adding things to the belt. He didn't though; he just put it all back. I guess everyone except Eric has spring fever.

I don't reply. I'm suddenly too tired to speak. This has been such a long day and it's not even mid-morning. I lean against my headrest, recline my chair, and close my eyes. I have no memory of the actual grocery store aside from the checkout, but this doesn't concern me. Remembering insignificant information is just one of the things my brain has forgotten how to do. If it's important, I'll remember. If it's important, I'll never forget.

"Tell me again—what did you say to that security guard?" Eric's voice interrupts the imagery dancing through my head. Again, I'd been walking through a forest. I could feel the dew on the leaves.

"What security guard?" I murmur, eyes closed.

"The one in Edmonton. When we went for breakfast yesterday morning before we drove home. Remember? We went to A&W after checking out? Hardly anyone ate."

"Oh, the young guy. I remember," I say with a yawn. The breakfast right after we argued about leaving our belongings in an unguarded truck in a dimly lit parking garage where a group of smokers lurked close by waiting for an opportunity. The breakfast right after the argument where Eric insisted that we needed food before we could leave, and I insisted that we could buy something on the road. And, not surprisingly, nobody ate because nobody was hungry so soon after waking. The breakfast right after that argument when Eric left me and the kids with no choice but to follow him when he stormed away from us. I didn't have my keys or I would have stayed behind, locked the children with me in the truck until he graced us with his return. Eric often leaves out significant facts in his version of a story. He remembers that no one ate, but he doesn't remember that was what I'd predicted during our argument, an argument that he has also conveniently chosen to forget even though I still feel its effects.

"I was buying food and I heard a big commotion behind me. When I turned around you were telling him something about us being in danger."

"No I wasn't." I open my eyes and look at Eric. Stare into him. "I was telling the security guard that there was something about to happen in the parking lot. There was a group of dangerous men conspiring."

"Right." Eric nods. "That's what you said you said."

"Yes. Because that's what I said. Did he say I said we were in danger?"

"No." He shakes his head. "That's what I thought you said. I can't remember if he came over to me or you brought him over or how I ended up talking to him."

I remember. I remember everything about that conversation.

"I was explaining to him that I thought someone should patrol the parking garage. He kept asking me what had happened and if I was okay. He wanted to know what I'd seen. He was nice but not helpful. He didn't get it. He wasn't listening." I glance at Eric. His eyes are on the road and his face bears no expression, as usual. "Then you walked up with the food and told me to go help the children. I took a tray and sat down. I'd been awake all night. I watched you talk with him for a while before you joined us. You were joking and laughing like old friends. You even clapped a hand on his shoulder."

"Yes. I explained that you were my wife and everything was fine but we were dealing with a health situation that was unravelling. I don't know why he believed me. For all he knew I could have been the reason you were in danger."

Again, I never said I was in danger. There is a distinction between me saying I am in danger and saying something looks dangerous, but I guess Eric doesn't see it. He rarely pays attention to the precision of my words. Not many people do.

"As I said, I told him there was something in the parking garage that needed attention, not that I was in danger. There was no commotion. We were having a conversation. And it's disappointing that he would believe I was fine just because you told him so when, as you say, you could have been the reason I was in danger. *If* I was in danger—which I never said I was."

"Right, right. Anyway, he just kept asking me if you were okay and if there was anything he could do."

Eric doesn't understand how frustrating this situation is to me, as a woman. I went to a male security guard with a problem, and my security was then handed over to my husband. Or the man who told the security guard that he was my husband, and then charmed him into walking away. What kind of security do women in this world have when a security guard concerned about a woman's wellbeing doesn't even follow up with her? And instead trusts the man who basically dismissed her to speak on her behalf?

"I think he was taken aback and didn't know how to respond," Eric says, as though reading my mind.

"I think basic training should cover active listening skills. And something about gender roles and not discriminating or being patronizing." I sound indignant. I am indignant.

"He was young," Eric says. He seems pleased with his analysis of the situation. I'm curious if the security guard did request that one of his colleagues patrol the parking garage, and maybe in doing so a crime was prevented. It's possible. I'm tempted to raise this point with Eric—that just because the three of us shared a conversation doesn't mean we each took away the same thing—but I'm also tired and ready to close my eyes again. I cradle my head against the seat-belt strap.

I wake to the click of the trunk being quietly closed. We're in the garage. Eric must have unloaded the groceries. I feel more refreshed after a catnap than I used to feel after a full night's sleep back when I used to sleep for a full night. I stretch, unlock my door, and walk through the garage, the backyard, and into the house.

"Sorry," I say softly. Eric is busy putting everything away. He doesn't notice me.

"Sorry that I didn't help bring everything in," I say louder. This time he turns, a broad smile that could be real or fake or something in between is plastered across his face. It's the smile he wears when he's hiding something, usually irritation.

"That's okay. Did you have a nice sleep?"

I nod.

"Maybe you should go lie down? Try to sleep more?"

I watch him empty bag after bag, folding each one neatly once he's finished with it.

"I need to draw."

He nods and exhales through his nose. Keeps unpacking groceries. I turn, walk out of the kitchen, and head towards my sketchbook. My outlet. My solitude.

Fifteen minutes later and I'm done my picture. It started out as a flower but then morphed into something resembling an onion bulb, which is still sort of a flower so I'm satisfied. It's the little details I've drawn that please me: a tornado, a spider, a sunrise, a crab. And, of course, the half-hidden word that ties it all together—the word that ties everything together. I leave it on the dining room table for Eric to discover. He won't comment, but the kids will. They love my art.

I'm not sure what to do next. I still feel tired but I don't want to sleep. Something bad might happen if I sleep. Plus, if I sleep now then I won't sleep tonight, again. Tonight will be better if I don't have a nap. I just need something to keep me busy. I just need to stop thinking so much. I pick up a book that I asked Eric to read, *The Best of Adam Sharp* by Graeme Simsion. I can't remember why I asked him to read it, but it has something to do with pining for the one that got away. And something else. If only I weren't so tired. Who did I think was pining, anyway? Eric? He's never pined for anyone. Am I pining? I can't recall. I sit in the living room and open the book, but the words are all jumbled. The sentences don't make sense and it's frustrating. Besides, I've already read this book. I start to pace the ground floor of our spacious two-story house, which I've recently noticed is partially shaped like a donut, so I can travel from room to room and pace in circles. The stairs are the hole in the middle, so I guess they're the Timbit. Oh! We should go to Tim Hortons and get Timbits!

"Eric?" I haven't seen him in a while but he's supposed to be here. He said he was working from home to keep an eye on me. Was he joking? Was he trying to trick me? Did he say goodbye, and I forgot?

"Eric?" I call louder. He's not on the main floor, so I climb the stairs, taking them two at a time, trying not to trip on the bridge. I hear water and nervously hurry into the bathroom. Eric stands in our glass shower, rinsing shampoo out of his hair.

"Hi," he says. "Everything okay?"

"Are you okay?" I ask. He looks okay but my eyes sometimes deceive me. They've been doing that lately: flapping a curtain when there's no breeze, mixing up the letters on our license plates, recognizing someone who turns out to be a stranger.

"I'm good," he says. And he is. He is so good. There is nothing more that I'd like to do right now than step into the shower with my husband and feel his hands wash my entire body. Not only will it feel fantastic but I also won't have to worry about slipping or doing anything dangerous to myself. I reach to take off my pants but he turns the handle and the water shuts off.

"Oh, I was going to join you." I pout.

"Sorry. I've got a call."

Of course he does. I forgot he was working from home.

"I was thinking we should go to Tim Horton's," I say hopefully.

"Sure, in about an hour, okay?"

I nod, gleefully watching Eric towel off.

"Would have been a nice shower," I say with the desiring eyes that he, and every other man I know, like so much.

"I bet."

He leans over to kiss me, and I lean in to make it more forceful.

"Rain check?" My husband is happy to be so adored. I nod and walk away. I am happy to leave him wanting more.

"Why is Suzie crying?" Eric demands.

"I turned off her movie," I say. Suzie wails on the couch beside me.

"Why did you do that?" he asks.

"She's had too much screen time." I yell over her sobs. Why is he doubting me? I've always been the one setting and enforcing screen time limits. I guess I just usually do it better because it doesn't usually end in tears. I guess I should have given Suzie five minutes instead of just shutting it down.

"Suzie, why are you crying?" I ask, leaning over her to speak directly into her ear. She is never this loud, and rarely this upset. She responds with incoherent preschooler gibberish, which is punctuated with shudders and gasps of air.

"I can't understand you until you calm down," I say, turning away. I stand up from the couch and walk to the kitchen sink to fetch her a glass of water. Eric stares at me, his furrowed brows focusing on my every movement.

"What?" I ask.

"Why did you turn off her movie?"

"Because she's had too much screen time. I just told you!"

He glares at me as he moves around to the front of the couch to sit beside Suzie, and starts to rub her back. I turn away from them to roll my eyes. He always jumps at an opportunity to be a hero. He has no idea how many tantrums and fires I've been putting out for the last decade while he's been at work, or how to do it properly and consistently to be effective. Her crying starts to subside, of course, and the too-noisy house becomes too-still. I put her cup on the counter, walk to the back door, and slide my feet into my Birkenstocks.

"Where are you going?" Eric asks. I ignore him as I step outside and half-slam the door behind me. I walk down the stairs and onto the concrete patio. I approach the grass and then slide my Birks off. I hear the door open and close behind me.

"Where are you going?" Eric repeats, louder.

"Nowhere." I scowl. I take one barefoot step onto the lush green grass, close my eyes, and tilt my head up towards the sun. Tentatively I place my other foot down, feeling the warm, soft blades of grass almost individually on the soles of my feet.

"What is going on with you?"

I turn to look at Eric. His head is cocked to one side and I can't read his expression. I think he might be more worried than annoyed.

"What do you mean?" I ask, and as I say the words I feel all kinds of emotions building up, wanting to be let out. Just like the tears that are starting to form behind my eyelids.

"You seem really... off, these days," Eric says, walking towards me. I notice that he leaves his sandals on when he gets to the grass. Poor Eric.

"I'm just tired," I say, waving one hand dismissively.

"No, it's more than that. What's going on?" He reaches out both hands to place on my shoulders.

"You wouldn't understand," I say.

There is a beat of silence. I assume he will leave me alone and walk back into the house.

"Can you explain it to me?"

That simple question somehow makes him so vulnerable and so trustworthy in my eyes. Sometimes he still surprises me, even though we've been together for almost twenty years.

"It's just—I have these urges for something I need and I need it right now. And often it's a colour. Like I need to feel a bright colour. But then if I feel too much brightness, I need dark colours. So right now we're on green grass. But when the green gets too much, I'll walk over here." I take three long steps until I'm standing on the concrete patio again. "Because this is kind of a grey-beige, so that's not as colourful. And it's rough, right? Hard? Not like the grass, which is so soft and comforting. The texture matters too. And the temperature—the grass is warm from the sun but the patio is cool so they're in perfect contrast for colour, texture, and temperature. Every time one of them gets too much, I can just step on the other one."

Eric looks at me with yet another look that I can't read. I think it's bewilderment.

"I'm sorry," he says. "I don't understand."

I knew he wouldn't. It was nice that he tried though.

"Where are we going?"

Eric takes his eyes off the road for a moment to glance my way.

"The hospital, Reesie. We're going to the hospital." I love it when Eric uses the endearing version of my childhood nickname, Reese. He must have something exciting planned.

"Oh, right, that's what you said. Then why are we headed towards the airport?" The highway in front of me is the one we took to pick his parents up when they came to visit us two months ago.

"We're not headed towards the airport."

I look again and realize that he's right. We aren't headed towards the airport. I wonder why we're going to the hospital. I hope nobody's sick.

"Where are the kids?"

"We just dropped Suzie off with Dana, remember?"

"Oh, yes. I got out to say goodbye when you wanted me to stay in the truck." Eric sure does like to be a controlling husband these days. Strange, because he's never been one before. I don't like it. Has he suddenly become jealous for some reason? Is it an Alberta thing?

"Yes," he says. It's as though all of his frustration and annoyance is contained within that one single word.

"And the boys?"

"Still at school. Dana will pick them up."

"Oh, that's good. I hope we won't be here long. Why are we going to the hospital?" I stare out the front window at the colourful road signs passing us by. The blue ones are my favourite, but every so often a bright yellow one sneaks up and catches me by surprise.

Eric turns to look at me, but doesn't answer. Or if he does, I don't hear him. We drive for a while before he exits the highway and we see the colourful building looming before us. He pulls into the parking lot.

"Okay, we're here."

I look at the sign that says "Emergency," and am disappointed to realize that we are, in fact, going to the hospital. I guess sooner or later I'll find out why.

## 7. Emergency Room

They're watching me. They're all watching me. Eric tells me they're not, they're focusing on their own problems, but I know better. They're staring. Staring at this ghostly figure with hospital gowns draped over her head to hide her ugly face, shielding it from them. I didn't want to come here. No, that's not true, I did want to come here, but that was because I thought Eric had a surprise. A party. The lottery. A baby. It's taking too long—Eric's scheme is too complex. Or maybe they've been telling me the truth and there really is no scheme. I don't know anymore. I don't want to be here.

The door opens forcefully and a South-Asian man walks into what they keep calling my room. He has dark brown skin and bloodshot green eyes. He is wearing a crisp white coat and black dress shoes. I feel shabby in comparison, even though Eric keeps telling me I'm beautiful. How can I be beautiful here in the Emergency Room? How can I believe anything my husband tells me when he keeps telling me things that are so obviously untrue? The brown man is not smiling, which makes me feel unsettled, but he is followed by the nice nurse who talked to us before. He likes us, likes Eric, likes that we're good people. He has a secret and I think it's that he's gay, but he keeps his secret buried. When we first arrived at the hospital I kept revealing everybody's secrets, but in the hours since, I've learned to bite my tongue. I could see in their eyes that I was right, but they refused to admit it, so they nervously dismissed my statements and added them to my list of delusions.

If we're not having a party then I think this must be something more. I think I've figured out something more. The meaning of Life. The reason there are so many coincidences. The truth behind the numbers. But I can't talk about it yet because I don't trust them, and they don't trust me.

Somebody starts talking and I'm not sure who because I'm looking at my feet. They're itching to move. The room is tiny, so I start to pace in spirals beside the bed. I like circles better than straight lines. One foot in front of the other, my right heel touching my left toe, as tight and coordinated as I can be, which is extremely tight and extremely coordinated because I am good at everything I do. The voice keeps going on and on and I don't know whose it is but I also don't care. Just wish it would be quiet. My crimson painted toenails look splendid against the navy sandal strap across my toes, it binds them all together as though they are five little monkeys jumping on the bed and need to be strapped in tight. Tight. That voice is growing stronger. Strap, strap, strap, stop it voice, belt, belts, diagonal belts, I said stop it, jacket, something, what's that thing, something, I don't know. You're too loud. You're too loud. You need to shut up I can't remember the word, there's something about the diagonal belts but I don't want to know.

All of a sudden the room is too quiet. My feet fall silent so I can lift my head up. There are three men staring at me. That's nothing new but their expressions are different from the familiar admiring glances I usually receive. Well, Eric of course is looking at me like he always does, but with a little more love and pride on his face. That's sweet. The nice nurse is looking at me like he's concerned. Why would he be concerned? Is something bad about to happen? Is it the party or the lottery or the baby? The brown man is looking at me with his red-green eyes and I have no idea what his expression says. Curiosity? Boredom? His eyes freak me the fuck out and I don't want to look into them again.

"What about a belt, Reesie, do you need a belt?" Eric says using an uncharacteristically tender voice. How does he know I was thinking about a belt? Can he read my mind now, just like I can read his? This is really getting intense!

"No, Reese, I can't read your mind."

He did it again!

"No, Reese, you're talking out loud."

No I'm not.

"Yes, you are."

No I'm not.

"Yes, you are."

Oh, really, Mr. Smartypants? Then what am I thinking now?

Eric sighs, then turns toward the strangers, and gestures at me with an upturned hand. He shakes his head. He's such a joker.

"See! Told you I wasn't talking out loud!" This time I do say it out loud. Oh, wait, that's the voice that wouldn't shut up. It was mine all along. Huh. I didn't recognize it. It has grown so powerful. So, I was wrong and Eric was right. Bizarre. That just doesn't happen anymore.

"Reese, this is Dr. Patel," Eric says, nodding towards the brown man.

"Hello," I say. My feet start to move in their familiar comforting circles again now that my head is firmly supported and doesn't need to change positions. I force myself to meet those scary eyes. This man's face is not unkind, especially now that he is smiling and now I can hear his voice. I can't hear his words, but it sounds like he's saying something gentle. A gentle giant.

"Your skin is so dark," I say. I take a second to drink him in when he pauses for me to answer whatever question he just asked. "I'm really light, even though I'm from South Africa, where a lot of people are really dark. Are you from South Africa?" My question sounds odd, but there are South-Asian people in South Africa too. He tips his head, and starts to scribble on the papers in his hand. He looks slightly amused, or maybe it's bottled irritation that I see. Compassion? It's hard for me to tell sometimes, especially with dark people. I grew up in Apartheid and we were all supposed to hate each other. Canada is different, I think. I look at Eric, who grew up in Canada but his parents are from Hong Kong. He is covering his face with both hands. He looks as pale as that ghost statue in the hotel. I wonder why. "My husband is dark too, even though he doesn't look as dark as you." I tell this brown man. "See his hair? And his clothes? We're like a yin yang except in reverse because the cold one is supposed to be the woman, right?" I drop my head down to look at my feet, images of yin yangs and peace signs and infinity symbols and arrows exploding like fireworks in my head, just like they have been in my sketchbook for days. I wonder if these men know that the dark, cold yin is negative and feminine, and the light, warm yang is positive and masculine. Probably not.

One foot in front of the other. These men don't make much noise for men especially considering there are three of them. Haven't found a topic they can agree on, I guess. No wonder women get a bad rap for being too talkative when all we're doing is bridging their silence gap. I'd like a good rap for a change.

"Just this morning or yesterday or maybe a month ago for all I know in this black hole room, it all clicked. It all makes sense," I say, keeping pace between my feet and words. It seems like they want something from me but I don't know what because they're not here for pleasure. They're good people. I can tell. The red eyes don't scare me anymore because this man seems gentle. Plus, Eric wouldn't let them do anything to me. Luckily he's here—he's always got my back.

"What makes sense, Charise?" This dark-skin-white-coat man furrows his brows.

Hmmm. Don't roll my eyes. Don't sigh. Don't show disrespect. Yet. But isn't he here to listen?

"All of it. Everything. Everything makes sense. Every single thing. Every single thought that enters my mind or thing I see or sound I hear or smell I smell." May as well spell it out for him and besides, the words go well with my feet. With the beat. He still doesn't seem to understand though. None of them do.

"Time's been funny lately, ya know? Like, I was doing everything and not rushing and it was like time had slowed to a thing. You know, like hickory dickory dock. Like a mouse. Not winded. Minutes slowed to hours. So much time I didn't have to yell. Or hurry them. No rush." It seems like as good a place to start as any. Time. Or colours. Or sleep. Or confidence. Or charisma. Pick a card, any card.

Eric's face is red, like when he drinks. Has he been drinking on the sly? I'd like some. His eyes have a strange bulge to them. He just can't take those bulgy eyes off me though. My husband, still so in love with me.

"Let's step back." I step back to demonstrate, and then forward, and then back again, rocking because it feels good, like when the kids and I play hopscotch, before I once again start to pace. "Do you know Daenerys? Targaryen? Or Margaery, something? I don't know her last name. She married that king so I guess it's Tyrell."

"She's talking about *Game of Thrones*," Eric says. Duh. Next he'll say he's reading my mind again. His voice sounds good though, almost like a backup singer except that we're talk-singing. It's fun! Like Eminem and Rihanna! I want to keep doing it. We rarely sing together and we never talk-sing. What's that word again for the talk-singing thing? Can't think of it. Move on.

"Margaery was the one with the grandmother. I had a grandmother. Margaery was obedient, clever, kind, and cunning. Sometimes selfish. Sound familiar, Eric?" I pause my talk song to give him a beat. My feet keep pacing while he takes too long to answer.

"Um, I guess," he says.

"But, Daenerys," I say quickly, and loudly, before he ruins our song. "She was the Mother of Dragons. Three dragons. I'm a dragon. A fire dragon. With three children. Just ask Eric, it's his zodiac."

I wait for Eric to fill in the chorus or the bridge or whatever thing it's called but he stares silently, clearly awed by my performance. I guess it's back to me, cleaning up after him as usual.

"So, I'm like both, right? The meek strong one who was killed, and the powerful fair Queen who walks through fire. Fire for me, no, but I love hot baths and I do that thing just like Julia Child with her hand in boiling water instead of the tongs."

I take a breath. The word comes back to me: rapping. I'm rapping. And I'm damn good at it for a middle-aged suburban mom. I keep going, but I decide just to talk this time. Slow my footsteps down.

"Plus the madness, right? The Targaryen madness? Something's happening, right, with the madness in me? I know, even though none of you are saying anything." I glare at Eric before I move one. "But the incest took a while to figure out because ew, gross, but not if we're reborn. What's that word when you live again after you die? Something about, re- something—"

The nurse mumbles but he's on the other side of my circle spiral so I can't hear him. I doubt it matters. He looks like a sheep.

"If we're that re-something then we're all related, right? We don't know who we're sleeping with from a past life. So, could be incest, right? But gross. Let's not think about it too long. Man, I feel like I have to explain everything to you guys."

The dark one nods his head along with my feet. So he gets the beat. Good. I like people who get the beat.

"Reesie, do you want to sit down?" Eric asks. I guess he wants in on my song now that he's seeing other people appreciate me.

"Nope." I shake my head a bit too fast. Dizzy. "But back to my grandmother. I miss her. She loved me so much. She tried to be good even though you know, South Africa. Apartheid. But she was good. We were scared. We were taught to be scared. Even after we came here we were scared. Check the locks, gotta make sure the door's locked, can't sleep with the window open even though we sleep better. We were so clueless about it all. Just like now, the news doesn't lie, right? We can trust the newspapers even if they're online? Hah!"

I walk a loop in silence, contemplating the McGill history course I took about South Africa. I learned far too many awful facts as an adult in Canada that I'd been oblivious to as a sheltered child in Germiston.

"So much propaganda," I say, pissed. "And they tell us to trust them. The newsmen, the government, the priests, the doctors, the self-professed experts like you." Here, I point at this brown man who commands authority because of a white coat. I should wear a white coat to be taken seriously. Not dismissed as an overly sensitive woman prone to overreacting or, worse, an overly sensitive girl. How come adults still call women girls? Like, fuck. My high school English teacher explained the difference decades ago but they still do it. "Back when she taught us about Madonna and the whore. All you people care about. She was so right." I take a breath. I need a new topic. A new rap. These men clearly can't be relied on to contribute. "Trust your gut. Listen to your spidey-sense. Follow your heart. But what if you've been suppressing your intuition for too long? What if it's stopped talking to you because it can no longer trust you? And then there's a sudden explosion and it all wants to—" I form my hand into a fist and raise it above my head. These men flinch, and the two I don't know take a step back, away from me. I release my fingers like a bomb exploding and purse my lips for my next act. "Boom," I whisper. Silence is more effective than rage. "Gandhi was a smart man. Must have had a smart wife," I sigh. "But McGill was fun, right Eric? Good thing '89 inspired me. Montreal. Mechanical Engineering. Who would have thought this good from that bad? If it weren't for that murderer we might never have met." The Montreal massacre happened on December 6$^{th}$, 1989, when a misogynist killed fourteen female mechanical engineering students at L'Ecole Polytechnique because he was "fighting feminism." It inspired me to study mechanical engineering, in Montreal, six years later. Eric and I met at McGill University in 1998. I look directly at him, give him that sexy smile he likes, and wait for him to sing.

"Yeah, Reese, McGill was great," he says slowly. Thanks for coming out, Eric.

"Well, what next then? Religion? I figured it out, by the way. It also took some thinking, but I got it. How they're the same. How to get that peace thing. I don't know if you guys would understand. It all makes sense but you guys just want the answers without having to do the work." I look directly at Eric here. "The priests. The priests. The priests are on fire. We don't need a lighter—let the motherfucker burn." I'm thinking in quotes now. I'd stop to ask if they noticed my clever wordplay, because unlike the song says, the roof is clearly not on fire and I said lighter instead of water, but they're not paying attention.Nobody's ever paying attention. I tell Eric to sub any word when he forgets the lyrics, but he doesn't listen to me. He's the musical genius. He doesn't think I know anything. About anything. He doesn't think my opinion is significant enough for him to pay attention. Which reminds me. "Did you know I'm Buddhist? I realized last week. It's been, what, a decade of yoga and meditation and all that stuff and finally, enlightenment. Daenaerys and Margaery with their reincarnation. But I'm not going vegetarian again. God, imagine? Cooking for all of you and separate meals for myself ? I do enough already. Jesus, I do more than enough already. Would it kill you to wash the dishes once in a while?"

I take a breath. Blow the air out as though it's smoke. I wish it were.

"What was the phone call about, Eric?" I say using my cold voice. He looks from me, to the men, and back to me.

"Do you need their permission to tell me?" My cold voice has heat.

"No, uh, what phone call?"

"The phone call. THE phone call. The good news phone call. The phone call you won't tell me about. The phone call that happened after the phone call about Jack that you also won't tell me about, not properly anyway. The writing competition phone call. The job phone call. The lottery phone call. The airport arrival phone call. The whatever-the-fuck-it-was-that-I-deserve-to-know phone call. Guessing, guessing, guessing, you always keep me guessing, keep me hanging on, keep me in the dark. The phone call on my phone that you took so I wouldn't make phone calls or write emails or texts or so you could look through it with your suspicious mind. Why is your mind so suspicious, Eric?" I say his name as a taunt. And then I remember something. "I liked the Nandy character in the waiting room, by the way. That was a nice touch. Chad could use acting lessons if he's going to keep playing that role."

He stares at me and then lifts up both hands to hold his head for a moment before wiping each one down his brow and the sides of his face.

"Who is Nandy?" the dark man asks.

"Her grandmother," Eric says, compressing his cheeks with his hands. "They were very close."

"Charise," the dark man uses his dark voice now, so he must mean business. I feel like I'm in trouble just by the way he said my name. "Can you slow down, please?"

"Slow what down?" I ask with an edge. I'm not in trouble. He has no authority over me! I don't even know this guy, how could he have authority over me? "What do you want me to slow down? Talking, walking, thinking, feeling, being, emoting, pulsing?" What the fuck is this stranger asking me to do? Whatever it is, I'm not doing it. I don't know him, why would I do something just because HE wants me to do it? I like what I'm doing.

"Slow down your words, please. Have you ever had a substance abuse problem?"

I start to laugh, and happy tears start to come, and before I know it I'm cackling so much that I can barely keep up with my beat.

"No, she's never had a substance abuse problem." Eric decides to speak for me again. That's fine, I'll allow it. It's an easy one and I'm already too busy juggling all of the hard ones that he keeps dropping.

"Were you ever abused?"

The question hangs between us. I simply shake my head. Doesn't this man know my family? Doesn't he know how lucky I've been? How could he even ask such a thing?

"Have you experienced this kind of excitement before? Or any severe depression?"

"No. Wait, yes. After the baby. The miscarriage." I look to Eric, who starts to elaborate on my behalf because it's obvious that I'm not going to. First pregnancy. 2005. Very upset. Yes, joined a support group. No major depression since.

"Hello? When Alex was a baby and wouldn't sleep," I say when he's finished. "And, you know, winter." I don't know if Eric even knows how down I get sometimes. In November. Or after I've failed. "But life goes on, right?"

"What about when you were at university?"

University? University was fun. I earned prizes and scholarships and excelled. Everybody loved me. Everybody wanted to be with me.

"I was on the Dean's Honour List," I say. "My GPA was 3.84. I got ninety-nine percent in BVP, do you know how hard that is?" The guy looks to Eric. Sure, let the men talk for and about me. Next they'll order my dinner.

"Boundary Values Problems," I say. "It is fucking hard."

"This kind of erratic behaviour typically reveals itself in someone in their early twenties," the dark man says, ignoring how smart I used to be.

Wait, did he just say that I'm too old to have fun? Or just too old?

"You're a funny man," I say, pointing an accusing finger at this dark skinned lab coat wearing expert.

"Reese, he's here to help you," Eric says. I give him a look. He knows the one.

"I don't need help. My soul compass is working again. It's stronger than yours, stronger than all of yours. Besides, these experts used to say everybody needed help. Took over from the midwives. Prescribed smoking to relieve stress. Gay people used to need treatment too, right doc? I bet he'll help me. He'll help me right into a lobotomy."

I take a gulp of air, and exhale in a seductive sigh. Time to turn from the madness. Flip to the charm. More flies with honey. But are they just going to stand here and watch me forever? Am I a performer now?

"I'm not actually a performer, you know. I'm a writer. First I'm a mom. I was an engineer, but now I'm a writer. Mom, writer, engineer, daughter, sister, teacher, therapist, chef, Madonna, whore. Many things to many people. I'm Wonder Woman. Just ask my keychain. But, you know, I might not be a writer. Have you seen my sketches, Eric? I think, maybe, I think I might be, I think I'm an artist." I say this last word breathlessly, like each letter is ten feet tall with brilliant lightbulbs exploding inside. Just like it looks in my head. Respect. "I wish you guys could see what I see, it's so fucking awesome. Mad genius, right?"

Still nothing from the peanut gallery. I'm beyond tired of this talk song thing. Maybe a different beat, a different tune. U2 comes to mind.

"This too shall pass. You know I just turned forty, right?" I don't bother to wait for a reply. "And forty is a special age, especially for a woman. It's when the very hungry caterpillar becomes a beautiful butterfly. The clever, diminutive sheep becomes a fearless, sexpot leader. All the years I've been learning and absorbing and learning and absorbing and a good little owl, and a quiet little owl, and a meek little owl, and a wise little owl. And now it wants out." I start to clap on this last word. "Out. Out. The dragon wants out. The wisdom. The power. The forty wants out. Bono wrote a whole song about it. '40.' Don't you guys know anything?"

My words are too fast. I can hear it, they're spiralling, like me. The dark man is still nodding along with my beat but now it's pissing me off so I stop. Not even tapping my toe. These guys are clueless. Even more than that, they're hopeless. And this is the guy who's supposed to help me? This clueless, hopeless, songless stranger? Hah. Whatever.

"So, is this party thing going to start or what? I don't want to leave Earth without my children." I look to Eric, panic-stricken. "We're not leaving without the children, right?"

He takes my hand, fuck, finally, and leads me to the cot thing they keep saying is my bed. As if. My bed is regal and it's waiting for me at home, with my children, which is where I should be. I climb up the single step to sit on it anyway. Feels comforting after so much walking. So much talking. So much so much so much.

The dark man starts to talk now, something about an inability to separate fact from fiction, paranoia, pressured speech, whatever that is. Whatever any of it is. He's using big words on purpose. Sounds phoney. These guys aren't art critics so how would they know? It's taken me decades to thicken my skin, but now I'm finally free, finally me, finally a dragon. I never knew I was one all along. They can criticize me as much as they want. They're not my target audience anyway.

The two men say something to me before they leave but I don't listen, just stare at the floor below my feet. I don't need to hear whatever agenda they're pushing. Eric and I are left alone again.

"So, is it a party?" I say quietly. I'm tired of waiting for Eric's surprise. It doesn't feel like it's a good one anymore.

"No, Reesie," he whispers. I look up. He's slumped in the reclining chair, head resting on his hands, elbows resting on his knees. So I can't read the expression on his face. Good one! It's easier for him to keep the secret if he doesn't look at me. I never knew my husband was such a good actor. I always thought he had too much integrity to be able to lie and sound convincing. I guess I was wrong. But he's starting to crack. Hopefully that means this will all be done soon and I can pretend it was worth waiting so long.

There is a knock on the door before it is pushed open again. The nurse is back. Wasn't he just here? Or was that yesterday? What day is it even? I am so fucking tired. Can't Eric just get this over with so we can go home?

"We need you to take this medicine," he says after a hushed conversation with my husband. It was hushed but it was also only three feet away from me so I caught snippets—big words like "psychiatrist," "mood disorder," and "anti-psychotic drugs," along with small ones like "sleep," "dinner," and "beds." Eric watches me with imploring eyes, waiting for my reaction. He stands behind the nurse, who holds two small cups out to me, one with pills and the other with water. I look at the cups and back to Eric. I raise my eyebrows wordlessly and Eric nods, so I reach for them, swallow the pills, wash them down obediently. The last few days have taught me that the only people I can trust are myself and my husband and if I have a moment of doubt then I must trust him above all else. A look of relief crosses both of their faces. Somebody takes the empty cups from me and does whatever it is you do with empty cups but that's too much for me to think about right now. I lie on my narrow bed and turn my back on the room. I feel Eric pull the thin blanket up to tuck me in, lean down to kiss my cheek, and lightly stroke my hair, but I stay quiet, staring at the wall. He steps away to dim the lights and then I hear him at the door, sharing more whispers and secrets with the nurse. I hear what sound like reassurances, which tells me that they're saying good things about me and I don't need to feel insulted or ignored. Their gentle voices calm me and I close my eyes. I stare into my dark eyelids, which become darker when I hear a click from across the room. Eric must have finished his conversation and turned the lights off. I hear the pleather arm chair squirm beneath his body as he sits down and props it into its reclined position. Within moments, the room is quiet, and all I can hear is the occasional intercom beep or wail from another patient down the hall. I turn over onto my left side, away from the wall, to reassure myself that Eric is still here with me and I'll be able to see him each time I open my eyes in this dark but not pitch-black room. He's here, asleep, like I knew he would be. Safe with that knowledge, I close my eyes again and this time allow myself to drift off. Finally, we sleep.

## 8. Manic Revelations

"Do you remember what Father David said when we got married?" I lean towards Eric to force eye contact. We're still in this room. Still waiting on something. Still running on empty. He looks exhausted, reclined in the puffy chair, next to the small table beside my bed. This emergency room is the jail cell in *Zootopia*, minus the glass.

"No. What did Father David say?"

"He told us to watch the sunset. He said to stay awake all night and watch the sunset. He said it would be the most glorious thing we would ever see." I'm not sure if he said the staying awake part, he might have said to wake up early, but since I have been staying awake all night for weeks, it feels like it makes sense.

"Sunrise." Eric corrects me gently.

"But we didn't, did we? We didn't watch the sunrise. We missed it. We were asleep. We've been asleep this whole time."

He nods. I don't think he gets it.

"Someone needs help. The kids. Are the kids okay?"

"The kids are fine, Reese. They're great."

"There's something wrong with Jack. Smell his breath. Something's rotting inside." I am overwhelmed by sadness. "Make sure he's okay?"

"I'll make sure." He looks serious. Like he's taking me seriously.

"It could be your Dad. Did you call him?"

"I called him, they're fine. They don't need help." His voice sounds calm, which reassures me. I don't think he's given up on me yet.

"Then it's someone else. Are my parents okay? What about my family? Someone at work?" There must be someone. There's someone I'm not thinking of. Who is it? It feels like when we go on vacation and I can't relax until I remember what I've forgotten to pack. I want that moment of relief, because once I know what it is then I'll know how to deal. If we don't know who we have to help then how can we help them?

"Everyone's fine." He moves beside me, wraps one arm around my shoulder.

"No. Someone needs help. If it's not family it must be work. Maybe that receptionist, she's always so gloomy. Or someone in the Toronto office. Maybe John. Maybe there's a problem with their baby. Or Michelle—she tries so hard and it's never good enough. Or it's someone else. Everybody needs help but there's somebody that you need to help. You."

I hear the urgency in my voice but Eric does not. I can't get through to him. He starts to rock and shush me. I don't think he's listening. Well, he's listening but he doesn't believe me. I've been trying to persuade him that something's wrong with me—something physical; I don't know what, but I have this feeling that I don't have much time and I can't ignore it. The tests came back clear so that's what he's choosing to believe. Doesn't he know that we're dying? Don't they all know that we're dying?

"We should go to Church." I pull away to look at him.

"What Church do you want to go to?" he says slowly, with uncharacteristic patience.

"I don't care, any one. But we need it. Remember how calm it was when we stopped at the Sports Hall of Fame on the drive home from Edmonton?" It was so bright and quiet and wholesome. It refreshed us after the frantic morning. "That was a Sunday and it felt like Church. It was so comforting. Maybe it doesn't have to be God, maybe we just need nature. Peace. Well, you need peace, I already meditate and do yoga. Maybe you should do yoga! But then maybe I need less peace. I need aggression, the opposite of calm. Tae Kwon Do! Or drums! Then we'd be balanced. We're already balanced together—you're so dark and I'm so light—but what if something happens to one of us? We need to be balanced within ourselves. Our own personal yin yangs, so we don't rely on each other. Something could happen to one of us." My words topple over one another, trying to escape. Everything is becoming so clear to me. It's extraordinary, and yet terrifying.

I pause to let Eric catch up. He wears a sad smile. As I stare into him, wrinkles literally appear on his face that weren't there moments ago.

"I want us to go on dates. A regular monthly date. Each month we take turns planning it and make it a surprise."

"Okay. We can do that."

My husband would agree to anything right now.

"You need to get your heart checked," I say with conviction.

"My heart's fine." His chin drops to his chest.

"It's not. There's something wrong. The doctor found something, remember?"

"But she referred me and I saw that specialist and he said there was nothing wrong, remember? I'm fine." He reaches for my hand.

"I don't think so. You often stop breathing when you sleep."

"That's not a heart problem."

"Then you need to get that checked too."

He doesn't know that when we die we will transcend to immortality. We will be reincarnated, but our new forms will remember this life. This is the offer that has been made to us here in the hospital, if not in so many words. I've been listening to the universe—by sticking together and refusing to turn on each other, we've proven our loyalty, proven our worth. But there are still obstacles, and one or both of us could still falter. Greed could win. We cannot die tonight in this hospital. We cannot choose our eternal happiness over the children.

"If we don't do this properly the children will be left alone. It's not just me being tested, Eric, it's you too."

He stares at me as though he's already figured this out and is relieved that I've finally caught up. I start to make even more connections and I gasp, covering my mouth with one hand.

"So that's why they had to get divorced! He's so rich and famous that it had to even out. Maybe they're not really divorced then. Maybe they're happy but it had to be a show. Or maybe he only became rich and famous because he caved when he was being tested. And then she had to leave. Because of what he'd done." Eric has no idea what I'm talking about. He doesn't know the celebrity couple or their story. That's okay, he doesn't need to.

I consider this and am struck with another thought.

"And that's why he had to die! Because they were one of the richest, most famous power couples and they had it all! She started a movement but people were too jealous to support her, because they had it all! And then he has this freak accident and she gets all this pity and becomes more popular and powerful than they ever were together. Do you think he's even dead? Was it all staged to help her cause? Or is there something more sinister? Did she have him killed? Or he wanted out because of her spotlight? Nobody can have it all."

The connections are actual lightning bolts in my brain. I can see them. I'm pacing again. Eric pulls me close, back to the bed, and I lean against his shoulder while he massages my back.

"I can make you happy or I can make you rich, but I can't make you both," I say.

His hand freezes and then continues to rub my back. He's rubbing in circles, so it feels right. I like circles.

"I have to tell you something," I say slowly. Tension hangs between us. His back stiffens.

"What?" His voice is a whisper. Like he's not sure he wants to know.

"I didn't do anything. Like anything physical. But a while ago I emailed Mark for his birthday and he said something about kissing me and I flirted back and it went too far. By email." My ex-boyfriend, once the love of my life, has always been a thorn in Eric's side. This guilty secret has gnawed at me for months and I'm glad to let it out. I'm not sure how Eric will react. I hope we'll be okay. I just want to tie up my loose ends in case something bad happens.

"Okay," he says slowly. "Too far how? Pictures?"

"No. Nothing happened. Just flirting. And reminiscing. Nothing real happened."

He exhales and murmurs reassurances into the top of my head. I enjoy it for a moment before pulling away. I don't know why he isn't annoyed. I would be. We are so different. I'm surprised and mildly disappointed. If he doesn't care about this secret, does he care about me?

"Do you remember what Nandy said?" I often think of my grandmother's wisdom in times of trouble.

He shakes his head.

"What it was all about—when she was dying. She said life was all about one thing."

"Okay. What was the thing?"

"I want you to remember."

"I don't remember."

"Think about it. It'd be better if you can remember."

"Just tell me."

I shake my head no and move on.

"Where are the children?" I know he's told me but I can't remember. I don't know why they're not with us.

"They're with Dana, remember? Our friend? Our kids go to school and play hockey together? They're fine. Don't worry."

"But are they scared? Do they know what's happening?" I don't know what's happening. I just don't want them to be scared. Or upset.

"They're fine." He pulls out his phone. "Dana sent me this picture. They're having fun."

And it's true, they are. I'm relieved and disappointed. Shouldn't they be a little bit concerned about me? He doesn't care, they don't care, does anyone care?

"We have to listen to Suzie," I say. "The youngest have the most wisdom because they haven't forgotten it yet. And pay attention to the trees. They were the first to talk to me."

I yawn and lie back on the bed, drained.

"You should sleep," Eric says softly. "I'll go get food and come back in a bit."

I bolt up to a sitting position.

"No, you can't go!"

"It's okay." He strokes my hair, easing me back down. "I'll be here when you wake up."

"It's not safe. We have to stay together. We're only balanced together!"

"It's okay. Remember I left to make those calls earlier and we were fine?"

I had forgotten, but he's right. And then I remember what I realized then: as long as we're in the same building we're okay. But I still don't feel better.

"What should I do if I need you and you're not here?" I say.

"Just think of something good."

"Like what?"

He pauses for a moment.

"The beat. Just think of the beat."

"Okay. That's good. Just promise me you'll think about it when you're gone."

He gives me a quizzical look.

"Think about what, Reese?"

I can't remember either. A moment ago it was so clear. Something about Nandy.

"The Mad Genius, Eric. Remember the Mad Genius?" It's not what I want him to think about, but I have to give him an answer. I don't want to look foolish.

"Okay. Mad genius. Got it."

He has no idea what I'm talking about, even though I've been talking about it for days. Genius is often mad. Genius is often crazy. It all makes sense. Finally. I'm starting to get ahead of myself again, starting to think too much, but then I hear it. The beat. The beat will save me. I've been tapping it out, pacing it out, singing it out, for days. Eric's been listening. I knew I could trust him. Suddenly I remember that the thing Nandy said wasn't when she was near death; that was when she kept talking about the darkness. The thing she said that I want Eric to remember was when we were having our picture taken and the photographer told us to say cheese. That's what he should know it's all about, because Nandy said so. But it's too late for me to tell him, he's already gone and I won't remember. But I usually remember, if it's important, and this is important. And he might figure it out. He said I should think of the beat and that was a good idea. Has he been paying enough attention? Will he see through my unintentional trickery? Was it even unintentional? Because she didn't say that was what it was all about, she just said it to make us laugh. But this whole time I remembered it wrong, which gave it a different meaning, so if I keep believing that's what she said, and that's why she said it, can that make it true?

I want to get up and pace again, so I lift my arm off my face and open my eyes only to discover that the room is now dark. My breath catches in my throat because I was not expecting darkness, but I force myself to exhale. Eric must have turned the light off. The simplest explanation is usually the right one. *This too shall pass.* I want to pace, but I am so tired, and so comfortable. It will please him if I sleep while he is gone. It will make the time go faster, so I don't feel so alone for so long. I roll onto my side, facing the wall, and close my eyes. Every few minutes there is a beep from a nearby machine, or an excited scream from one of the other inmates that startles me awake, but I am tired enough to fall right back to sleep by focusing on my breath. And thoughts of my children. And images of trees. I am just so tired.

## 9. Poor Judgment

I sit on the edge of this bed, tapping my pinkie against the mattress. My legs want to stand and walk to the sink, but I've already investigated there. I've also already arranged the objects on the counter beside the sink to be functional and artistic. Beauty is better than practicality, but both together make the perfect combination.

"How long are they going to keep us here?" I say, and the words of Bono come to mind, "How long to sing this song?" Eric looks calm and handsome sitting on the armchair with his feet propped up and his eyes closed. They open at the sound of my voice.

"I thought you were asleep," he says.

"How could I be asleep? Isn't it the middle of the day?" I ask. The overhead light is off, but a small beam glows in the corner of the room. "Didn't we just sleep all night?"

I have no way of knowing the time. I handed my phone over to somebody long ago, although I don't remember who. Maybe Ryan, the nice nurse, or Jay, the equally nice and not as serious nurse, or maybe Eric. Or a doctor. I don't know. I just know that I have no phone, no watch, and this room has no windows so there isn't natural light to trigger my body clock. I've just woken up feeling like I've slept a full night, like I often did when one of our babies finally slept a full five hours. Once, I woke up so refreshed at two o'clock in the morning that I began to iron all of Eric's dress shirts. I was wired after having been sleep deprived for so long. It was exhilarating. I feel that way now.

"It's ten." Eric says after checking his phone. I thought he wasn't supposed to have his phone either, something about the machines. But I guess not. I guess it's just me. I don't know why. Who can remember everything they've said?

"Wow, we slept in!" I can't remember the last time I slept until ten. No wonder I have so much energy.

"No, Reesie, it's ten at night."

What? That doesn't make sense. I try to figure it out but my brain is so confused.

"What time did we go to sleep?"

"You fell asleep after dinner. Around seven."

I nod and hop to the floor. The cool tiles feel good on the soles of my feet. Steadying.

"So, I've been asleep for three hours."

Eric nods. His mouth is stretched taut in a frustrated grin. I guess he'd hoped I would sleep all night.

"This room is a prison cell." I look around as I pace, taking in the pale green paint, weird wall that looks like a garage door, and lack of a window. Fresh air would feel so luxurious right now. Eric's eyes follow mine and it's as though he's seeing everything for the first time.

"Yeah, it kind of is," he says. For some reason his affirmation floods me with relief. I'm not the only one who sees the room for what it is. My observation is valid, and won't simply be dismissed, like everything else I've said in here.

The door opens, as though on cue. A brown man wearing a white lab coat enters the room, with Ryan close behind. He looks familiar but I can't place him. There is a woman in a bright floral dress and another white lab coat who follows both of them. Ryan says something about my husband being concerned about me, which doesn't sound right. What does Eric have to be concerned about? I think the dark man might be the doctor. He starts asking me questions and I answer, with no idea what I'm talking about. I know I'm babbling, but I can't seem to stop. I just want to go home. Am I saying the right things so I can go home?

"You were pacing the last time I saw you. Do you always pace like this?" the doctor asks.

"Like what?" I look at my feet and watch as they spiral in and out, one foot in front of the other. When I get to the middle of the spiral-circle, my feet decide to turn around and walk from the inside out again. When the circle gets too big for this space, they turn back and shrink in on themselves. My feet are so clever.

"She doesn't usually pace," Eric says, speaking on my behalf after I've been silently observing for too long. How would he know, just because he doesn't see me pace? I pace all the time, especially when I'm on the phone, which is usually when he's at work. Does he think I'm a tree in the forest and I make no sound when I fall simply because he's at work?

"I pace when I'm on the phone. Or trying to think. Or trying to calm down." They're not looking at me. They don't care. "Wait, are you my doctor too?" I ask the woman. She hasn't said anything. Even when I complimented her dress she just chuckled. I'm not sure why someone would chuckle at a compliment.

The man stares at me with his green bloodshot eyes. From the expression on his face it seems like he's asked me a question and is waiting for my response. I wish I knew what to say.

"I've noticed that my nails are splitting. See?" I lift up my hand to show him. The nail on my ring finger on my right hand has started to split, and the middle finger nail looks like it's trying to decide whether to follow suit.

"No matter what I do, for weeks, it keeps splitting. Do you think it could be related to why I'm here? In Edmonton I thought I was pregnant but maybe not. Maybe it's menopause and the hormones are wreaking havoc on my body and making my nails split and my insomnia worse. I usually can't sleep before I get my period so it could be related to hormones," I say, pausing to take a breath. I'm sure this man will have an answer for me. I just wish I could get my nails to stop splitting.

The doctor, the nurse, the woman, and my husband all look at me as though I'm crazy. No, something worse than crazy: irrelevant. As though my words are meaningless, and my thoughts bear no weight at all in this conversation. All I am doing is wasting everybody's precious time.

"You should ask your family doctor about your finger nails." The doctor stands up—wait, when did he sit down and where did he get the stool from? Do I have a secret stool closet hidden in my prison room? He walks out with his coat tails and entourage following. Ryan the nurse turns at the last minute.

"I'll be right back, guys," he says, looking directly at Eric. Eric nods his assent and leans back against the headrest of the chair. I can't tell if he's wearing a look of concern or disgust. I continue to pace and the beat comes almost instantly. I want to sing but it doesn't seem like Eric's in the mood for it. Still, the words want out.

"Did you check with your parents?"

"Mmm."

"Everybody's okay?"

"Mmm."

It feels like we're doing a duet, working in time with each of my footsteps. I wonder if Eric's doing it intentionally because he knows I like it.

"How 'bout my mom?"

He opens his eyes, looks at me, takes a deep sigh, and nods his head. I guess he wasn't doing it intentionally.

"Did you talk to Dana recently? Are the kids okay?"

He doesn't answer, simply stares. His expression is turning stony. Time to switch topics.

"I've been thinking that our forties are for our careers," I say. He tilts his head. An invitation to continue.

"I've been writing my book for ten years. I have to finish."

Eric nods.

"But I don't know if I can," I say. This thought makes me tear up. "I need help."

"Okay. We can get you help," he says. I feel instant relief and I smile at him with gratitude.

"And I think you could do really well in your career if you focus instead of getting lazy."

He frowns, clearly offended because he thinks I'm saying he's lazy. And he says *I'm* too sensitive.

"Like, if you seek new challenges. Keep asking for more." I have to concentrate very hard to get the right words out, so I am slow. And a bit slurred. "They obviously like you and want you. But you're starting to get bored. Soon you'll wonder if the grass is greener."

Eric props a hand under his chin and looks to the ceiling to consider my analysis. Then he looks back to me.

"That's probably true."

"I think you said they've been really supportive about this," I flap my hand at the room to imply that they've been supportive about whatever it is that's happening these days. "I think you should recognize how good you have it. Figure out how to make it better so you stay—" I can't think of the word. Something about success. My head is so heavy.

"Engaged. Fulfilled." Eric nods, staring into my eyes while clearly thinking about something else. He looks not happy, exactly, but something. Better than he's looked since we got here anyway.

"But we've got to get rid of that carpet," I say. "The runner, upstairs. It's dead. It's poisoning us. We'll all sleep better when we can breathe."

The look on his face returns to one of resignation. No, it's a look of defeat. Weary defeat. What did I do now?

Ryan walks into the room. He starts to talk but I tune him out because I don't really care what he says and he's talking to Eric anyway. And I'm listening to my thoughts, which *are* important.

"I need the bathroom."

Both men turn in my direction. Neither one looks happy to be interrupted. I went to the bathroom earlier, it was just down the hall. I could go by myself if they'd let me, but of course they won't. Of course they claim to want what's best for me even though I've been going to the bathroom by myself for decades.

"I'll let you know once I've heard anything," Ryan says before smiling at me and walking out. He leaves the door open, which is a pleasant change. Somebody screams down the hall and Eric startles and then looks to me for my reaction. I smile.

"Maybe they really need the bathroom," I say. "Or maybe they won the lottery."

"Maybe," Eric says slowly. He looks like he's trying to figure out if I'm joking. I don't know the answer to that. "Okay, let's go."

He keeps one hand on my elbow as he guides me down the hall, the way he did in the hospital after we had the babies. Then it hits me. We are in a hospital! Maybe that's just what people have to do with people in a hospital, hold onto their elbows! Maybe it's a rule. But why am I here again? I thought we were coming for a surprise.

"You know, I'm starting to think there isn't going to be a party," I say after Eric has closed the door to the bathroom and started to clean the toilet seat. I've been reluctant to say these words out loud. He washes his hands and looks at me.

"No, Reese, there's no party. You're not pregnant. Nobody won the lottery. We're in the ER to figure out what's wrong with you. Dr. Patel is your psychiatrist."

*Wrong with me?* His words scare me, so I repeat my go-to mantra: *this too shall pass.* I know that I'm slipping. I've known that all along. Something is happening and I don't understand. I need another mantra. I know: *trust Eric.* I silently say these words as forcefully as I can to remember: trust yourself, but if you and Eric don't agree, trust Eric. He is the one person you can trust in this building full of strangers trying to tell you what to do. Trust Eric.

"What's wrong with me?" I ask after a few calming breaths.

"That's what we're trying to figure out."

Well, that just sounds absurd. Nothing's *wrong* with me. I'm just not sleeping well. And my nails are splitting. So that's what's wrong with me, but I don't need a hospital for that. Unless I am pregnant, and he's not telling me because there's a problem. I really felt pregnant in that hotel room in Edmonton the other day. Could he be keeping that a secret from me? Maybe they're all worried about telling me the truth because they think I can't handle it, because it devastated me when I miscarried our first baby. Does he really think I haven't grown after twelve years and three amazing children? Does he really think he's doing this to protect me, because I can't handle it? I'm reminded of Ani DiFranco asking, "Am I a kitten, stuck in a tree somewhere?"

"Do you need help?" Eric asks.

I shake my head no. Exhaustion hits me again.

"Okay, I'll wait for you in the hall." Oh, he was talking about going to the bathroom. No, I don't need help going to the bathroom.

"Do you think that's allowed?" I ask as the door closes behind him. I don't want to get in trouble. I don't want to have to stay here longer. I use the toilet and wash my hands quickly, eager to get out of this room before they notice Eric lurking outside the door and start asking him questions. I find him pacing the small space beside the washroom. He paces in straight lines. He takes my elbow again and starts to guide me back to my room. I feel anxiety building in my chest.

"Can we just stay out a minute?" I ask, my eyes pleading with his. Being locked in that windowless, airless room after learning that there's no good news and possibly some bad news is just too much right now.

"Out where? Here?" Eric asks, glancing up and down the hall.

"Anywhere. I just need space to breathe."

"Okay," he says. "Let's walk."

I link my arm through Eric's, which is propped at his side. It looks like a triangle with a hole in the middle, strange that I've never noticed that before. But then shapes have made themselves more obvious lately. Of course his arm makes a triangle, triangles are the strongest shape and we are the strong core of our strong family. Things keep making sense. We are such a great team.

We walk down the hall, past my door, around a corner, and alongside the nurses' station. Ryan sits at the desk. He raises his eyebrows at Eric as we approach.

"She wants to stretch her legs," Eric says over my head to Ryan. I'm lucky that Eric is here to speak for me and take care of me. I shouldn't doubt him. He wants what's best for me. He'll do what's best for me. Surely he knows I'm not an invalid and I can handle it, whatever it is. *Trust Eric.*

"Okay." Ryan nods. "Just to the end of the desk and then back, please."

I slow my pace, reluctant to have to turn around in the few small steps that separate us from the end of the desk. Despite my efforts to drag it out as long as possible, we reach our invisible wall too quickly and Eric turns towards me. He then guides me to turn around.

A teenager approaches who is wearing the same hospital pyjamas as me—when did I change into hospital pyjamas?

"Where is my outfit?" I whisper.

"What outfit?" Eric asks.

"The one I was wearing." For the party. Or the baby. Or—something. "I loved it."

"You were wearing pyjamas and a piece of cloth draped around you. It looked like rags."

"Where is it? It was special! Why am I in hospital pyjamas?"

I don't want to offend the approaching hospital pyjamas-wearing person who must also be a patient, so I drop it. As he gets closer I notice his pant legs are too long. I look at my own and see that they are rolled up at the bottom and down at the waist. I step forward to meet him in the middle of the gap between us and I kneel down to roll up his pants, making neat little cuffs.

"Reese, no," Eric says behind me. I look over my shoulder to see that he is scowling at me. One hand covers his mouth and the lower half of his face.

"What?" I say. "He'll fall." I don't understand what Eric's problem is.

The teenager stops walking, glances down, and switches legs for me to roll the second one when I've finished the first. His hands are close to my face and I stare at his fingernails, which are longer and more pointed than anyone's I've ever seen. They remind me of the devil. I hope he's not the devil. My heart skips a beat at the thought but luckily I'm finished so I step back quickly, as if licked by a flame. Eric guides me back into my room with a little too much pressure on my arm.

"Why are you rushing me?" I say. "I don't want to be in here."

"Some of the people out there are dangerous! Don't you hear everybody screaming?" Eric sounds a little frantic.

I listen for a moment.

"No," I say.

"Earlier. It's late now—everyone's asleep."

Something's almost connecting. Didn't he say we're in a psych ward? Or the Emergency Room for a psych ward? Don't crazy people get louder when it's late? I can't think it through.

"I heard yelling before. I thought people were celebrating."

"Nobody was celebrating, Reese. This is a psych ward."

Aha! It *is* a psych ward.

"So, why were they yelling?"

He shrugs his shoulders slowly, with intention.

"That guy whose pants you just rolled up had pee all down his leg," he says.

"What? No he didn't. His pants were dry."

"No, they weren't. You shouldn't do that to a stranger anyway."

"His pants were too long. He was about to fall." Why is this so difficult for Eric to understand? I've been rolling up pant legs for over a decade, ever since Alex started wearing pants. It's usually my own children's pants, but sometimes it's not. Moms help other kids when they need help.

"He was a big kid. He didn't pee his pants." I say. I was a lot closer than Eric and didn't see or smell anything. And lately my sense of smell has been stronger than it's ever been in my life. All of my senses, in fact. "You must have seen a shadow."

Eric doesn't answer me, just helps me up onto my cot-bed and covers me with the thin blanket Ryan brought in earlier. He gently pushes me back until my head rests on the flimsy pillow. He kisses my forehead.

"Get some sleep, okay?"

Oh sure, because it's just that easy. Especially now that he's gone and got me all agitated, and now that we're locked back in this room. I lie in the darkness with my eyes wide open, try to breathe to calm down. I wait. For what, I don't know.

## 10. Demanding Trust

"They've got a room for you," Eric says. He starts to pack my snacks, book, and random trinkets I've left lying around this prison cell.

"What?" I sit up and rub my eyes. I think I was just about to fall asleep. The fluorescent lights burn, making this stark room feel more austere. "I thought they said I had to go for an MRI."

Eric stops moving, stands up straight, and turns to look at me.

"You went for the MRI. You don't remember?"

I shake my head. He starts to describe it. Middle of the night, they wheeled me in semi-conscious, he was awake and looked at the images with the technician.

"I guess I was asleep." A vague memory of being woken up appears in my fragile mind. "I think I remember lying down and being slid into the machine."

Eric stares at me with a look that's difficult to read. Either concern, disbelief, or maybe he's just worn out. That's the look. Exhaustion.

"Don't leave me, okay?" I ask.

"I'm not going anywhere," he says. That breaks the spell. He squeezes my sweater into the bag and zips it closed.

"No, like, don't leave me. Don't end our marriage." I have this overwhelming feeling that he is done. That this is all too much. He raises his eyebrows and shakes his head, smiling at me.

"I'm not going anywhere, Reesie," he says. Just then the door opens.

"Are you ready?" a voice asks. I don't look up because I don't want them to see the tears in my eyes.

"Yes," Eric says. He picks up the bag with one hand while reaching to help me down from the bed with the other. I slide into my flip flops, which are conveniently on the floor beside the bed.

"Did you bring my flip flops?" I ask. I don't remember packing anything but Eric has this bag full of stuff. Where did it come from? He holds my hand tightly and guides me forward. I reach the door and see a wheelchair in the hall.

"I can walk," I say to whoever is listening. Apparently no one is because I am directed to sit and they won't take no for an answer. Okay, so I get a ride. I've never been in a wheelchair before. At least I don't think I have. It feels new. I reach for the wheels, but somebody tells me to sit back. I turn to see a stocky brunette standing beside my wheelchair. She's wearing a uniform. I think she's a security guard. The wall behind her is moving, sliding away from us as though we're on a soundstage, pretending to be driving a car.

"Look at the wall," I say to Eric, pointing. He glances at it and then back to me with a look of indifference, as though he walks past moving walls every day.

"Look, Eric. It's moving!"

"The wall's not moving, Reese. We are." He points forward as though asking me to face forward, so I do. Sure enough, we're moving.

"I guess I need more sleep," I say. I feel like it's a joke but nobody laughs. I turn back to the woman again.

"Hello. We weren't introduced. My name is Charise."

"Hi Charise," she smiles. "My name is Christine."

"It's nice to meet you, Christine." I'm proud of my adult-sounding conversation. I try to hold onto this normal feeling.

"It's nice to meet you too," Christine says.

I'm tempted to ask her if she comes here often, but I get the feeling that my sense of humour is no longer appreciated.

"How long have you been working here, Christine?" I ask. I have to remember to repeat her name to remember it. I'm sure I'll see her again and people always feel good when their names are remembered.

"Oh, about five years now." We've reached the elevator bay so we stop and someone pushes the button. Eric stands on the other side of me, glancing around as though to check if people are looking. I don't know why he thinks we're so entertaining.

"I guess you must like it," I say. This conversation is going nowhere.

"I do. The staff here are great."

"They seem great!" I say, too excited. I've only met a couple of nurses and that dark doctor who kept tapping his foot to my beat while he cross-examined me, but they did seem nice.

"You know, my husband can take me wherever we're going. You don't have to come with us," I say. I'm sure she's busy.

She smiles a thin-lipped smile to avoid an awkward response.

"Oh," I say. "You have to take me there."

Christine nods. I'm not offended. The elephant's only awkward when we don't address it.

"I see. Okay." The elevator arrives, so somebody starts to push me again.

"Where did you work before here, Christine?"

"Well, I'm from Ontario originally."

"Oh! So are we! Where in Ontario?"

I think she says Thunder Bay but it might be Fort Erie and those are two very different places and I know nothing about either one since I'm from Toronto and even if I did my adult-conversationing is starting to wear me out.

"Do you still have family there?" I ask. It's my final attempt to keep this thing going. She says yes and starts to elaborate and thank goodness because I can't do this anymore. She is lovely and I want to keep talking to her forever, it's just that I'm not good at forever right now. I sit facing forward—catatonic—and enjoy the comfortable silence that develops between us once she stops making words.

"Okay, we're here," Christine says. She flashes her pass in front of a keypad and the door opens, which feels like déjà vu because didn't she already flash her pass in front of a keypad and the door opened? I want to ask, but not if it makes me look more crazy. And I don't want to talk about the past. It's just a bridge we burned down. Eric keeps saying so in that Lightning Tent song he keeps singing. There is too much future inside this new door. A long hallway. An exercise bike! Laundry machines. The smallest fish bowl I've ever seen and a real live fish swimming in it. A huge window way, way down there. A nurse sits behind a desk waiting to greet us. Behind her are several colourful signs on the wall. One says, "Today is Thursday," with a big happy face. But didn't we come to the hospital on Monday? Did four days pass in that ER? Everyone else does all the talking and then it's time for the nurse to search my bag and it's time for Christine to go and I'm sad that she's leaving when we were just getting to know each other.

"Make yourself comfortable and we can go over the rules again when you're ready." The nurse lady says. What rules? Did she just tell us rules? I'll have to ask Eric because we're being led into a huge room with a single bed covered in a pink blanket. Wait—why am I walking? What happened to my wheelchair? Didn't they say I needed it? Is something wrong with my legs and they haven't told me? I reach for Eric and lean against him for support. He guides me to the window bench and helps me to get settled. It's a dreary day outside, which is strange for Calgary. I see houses in the distance, but directly in front of me is the hospital rooftop. Grey clouds chase each other in the sky above. A storm is coming. This will be a good spot to watch it.

"Is today Thursday?" I pull my legs up underneath me on the cushion.

"No, it's Tuesday," Eric says. "Why?"

But if today is Tuesday, then that means—

"We just got here yesterday," Eric says, as though he really can read my mind. I didn't think I'd lost four days, but it also doesn't make sense that we've been locked away for so long and it's only been one day. Twenty-four hours. And no end in sight. How am I ever going to survive in here if it takes an eternity to get through a day?

# 11. Confusion

"You need to sign this form." The nurse hands me a piece of paper that I can't read. I try to decipher the letters and spaces, but nothing makes sense. It's the end of my first day in the psych ward, and it has been a long one. I was okay until it was time for Eric to leave. I even joked about this being a low-budget spa for moms who need a break. But the bubble burst when he had to go. When he left me alone.

"It says you're here on an involuntary basis and will stay here for up to thirty days based on our assessments," the nurse explains.

My heart starts to pound. I feel cold sweat on my back. I have no way of knowing if what she's saying is true. I have no way of knowing if anything they say here is true.

"I'm sorry," I say. And I am. "I don't understand. Why does it say I'm involuntary when I came here voluntarily?"

She rambles off an explanation that she herself does not seem to understand. I don't want to sign something that says I'm involuntary, because that's bad. It would mean I'm bad, like they're saying I'm refusing to comply, when all I've done so far is comply. How can I be refusing to comply if I'm complying to sign the form that says I'm refusing to comply? I feel like I'm being coerced. I feel like I need a lawyer present, or at least a witness.

"If you'd prefer, we could wait until tomorrow when your husband is here," the nurse says after I've awkwardly stared at the paper for too long.

"Is that okay?" I look up desperately. "I'm having trouble focusing. And he's a lawyer, so I don't ever sign anything without him reading it first." Why didn't they have me do this form thing when Eric was here?

"That's fine." She grabs the paper from my hand and drops it in a folder which she quickly snaps shut. Relieved, I stand and walk back to my room. I am asleep within minutes.

There is a knock on the door and a moment later Eric walks through it and into my room. I'm sitting where he left me last night, on my window seat, trying to read a book. The words are all jumbled.

"Reese, what happened?"

He sits down beside me, hugs me, and keeps his arms resting in my lap.

"What do you mean?" I ask. There are so many things that have happened, which one is he talking about?

"They said you wouldn't sign a form."

"Oh, yes!" I beam. I am so proud that I waited for him to read it before I would sign it. "I didn't understand it and she couldn't explain it. I thought you should read it first."

"That's good," he says, using a tone that implies it is anything but good. "But, I think what you need to do for now is really listen to what they say and do what they want you to do."

I stare at him, watching his loyalties divide.

"I *was* listening. The form didn't make sense. She wanted me to sign that I was an involuntary patient so they could hold me for thirty days. But I came here voluntarily, so how am I involuntary? And what are the implications of me saying that I am involuntary? Can they take away my rights? Isn't signing something an indication of willfulness? Of voluntariness? I asked her to explain it and I kept trying to understand, but it made no sense. She didn't seem to understand it herself."

"Yes." He nods. "I saw the form. It doesn't make sense. I don't understand it either."

My relief lasts but a moment before it turns to irritation. Eric prattles on about how I need to be obedient and prove I'm listening, and how the staff knows what's best for me and doing what they say will show them I agree. I tune it all out. I'm not a child. How could they know what's best for me when they don't even know me?

"Don't you want to go home?" His question breaks through my thoughts.

"Of course. Are you taking me home?" My heart skips a beat. Could it be possible?

"No." Eric shakes his head before resting it in his hands. "Reese, just do what they want you to do, okay?"

I nod. Take doctor's orders. Listen to the nurses. Obey, without question. Sign forms that don't make sense. Trust everybody above myself. Suppress my questions, thoughts, and instincts. No problem. My throat grows hot and tears prick the backs of my eyes.

"How are the kids?" I ask, desperate to know because they're all I've been thinking about.

"They're good," Eric says after exhaling. He tells me about play-dates and sleepovers and it all sounds like a party—great for them, sad for me. What if they want me to stay at the hospital because it's more fun without me? What if they never want me to come home?

"Your mom arrives tonight," he says.

"What?"

"Your mom arrives tonight. Remember? I told you she's flying in."

My mom hates to fly. Hate is too mild. She will not fly.

"She doesn't fly," I say.

"She does now." It's clear from Eric's tone that he no longer wants to discuss this. No longer wants evidence of my confusion. I want answers, but I don't want to make him more frustrated with me. He looks tired. *Suppress.* He lies on the window bench and pulls me down, so that my head rests on his chest. We've done this dance so many times over the years that of course I know what happens next. He will be asleep in less than a minute, and I will relax, listening to his heartbeat. We will stay this way for a short time, until the pressure of his chest against my ear starts to hurt or until I get antsy with thoughts about what I could be doing instead, and then I will get up. He won't notice, he will continue to nap for however long it takes before he has enough energy to wake up. No matter how much he sleeps it never seems to be enough. No matter how much I'm awake it never seems to be enough. We are a perfect complement, like the yin yang I kept doodling last week. That reminds me, he brought me a sketchpad. Finally, I'll have something else to do in here, something that I choose. Something that I love. I don't know how long I'll be in this place, but I know I'm going to need something to pass the time besides pacing in spirals.

# 12. Advocating

"Charise is an engineer, a wife, a mother. She's intelligent, logical, and more than capable. She's not like the other patients in here." Eric's voice carries and the volume increases with each word. His tone is meant to admonish my nurse. He is angry and frustrated. I feel loved. I've been here for three days and of all of the feelings I've had, loved is the best.

We stand in the hall. At least, he stands in the hall. I stand just inside my doorway, as close to the hall as I can get. Watching Eric foam at the mouth, I feel proud and entertained. It can be fun to watch him in full force. Plus, it's nice that he's back on my side instead of doing his charming act for the staff. Maybe it's because it's a nurse, not a doctor, and she's not particularly attractive. Either way, he's on my team, at least for now.

My nurse is stern and has likely seen it all, so she is not reacting the way Eric hopes. He's used to getting his way when he puts his foot down. He leans in, furious, pointing his finger at her, accusatory, and yelling louder than any of us crazy patients at the moment. If I was behaving like him, I'd be put in what they call a "high-observation room," with nothing but a mattress on the floor. They'd take away my bedside table filled with books, toiletries, drawing implements, snacks, and other comforts from home. They'd force me to hand over my clothes (the ones I couldn't wear in the ER but was given back when I was transferred here) in exchange for a gown. By high-observation they mean no-privileges. No respect. No dignity. When I first arrived on the ward, I thought it was the craziest of crazies that wore gowns, but then I figured it out—they're just the least obedient.

It is for exactly this reason that Eric is so upset: my clothes have been taken away. And all my stuff. And my dignity. When he left yesterday evening to go home to our children and my mother, I was in a bright, spacious room with furniture. A bed frame. A window seat, even. The tulips he'd brought me. Magazines. Moisturizer. When he arrived this morning, I'd been moved to an empty room with a lonely mattress. Even my hairbrush and toothpaste were confiscated. So was my clean underwear. I looked a wreck—crazy.

"What happened?" he said, sitting beside me on my mattress on the floor.

"They had to move me," I said, waving a hand dismissively, trying to downplay it.

"But, why?" He looked around. "Where's your stuff ?"

"It's fine," I said. "Just the nurses doing their jobs."

I don't know why I was moved, but surely they must have a reason. I couldn't care less about sleeping on the floor, although I would like my tulips. Eric was taken aback. I saw it on his face. I see too much on people's faces, but his reaction confirms that I'm not always wrong.

My nurse calmly waits for Eric to get the anger out of his system. I am so moved by his loving speech that I have to bite my lip to keep from reacting. After all, it was my reacting that got us here. Lucky for me, I have someone like him to advocate on my behalf. I wonder what happens to the ones who don't. The ones no one listens to.

"We had to move her because of her actions last night. She tried to escape, so she had to be put in a room with surveillance." The nurse is calm, cool, and collected.

Eric turns to look at me, baffled.

"You tried to escape?"

That's not the right word. I just followed the numbers on the doorplates down the hall, and each one told me something new. The patterns kept telling me to go on. Until I got to the end.

"I didn't try to escape. I know there are two sets of locked doors." I look at Eric with pleading eyes. I'm not an idiot, Eric, you know this about me. Stay on my team. Please.

My nurse has less patience for me. She won't listen to me like she listened to Eric.

"It says in your file that you tried to escape," she says. She looks at her wristwatch. "That was the reason for the room change."

"I thought they might let me out if they knew I was ready to go home. I keep asking when I can go and no one gives me a straight answer. I thought I just had to prove I wanted it. I just had to act. Remember that line from *The Last Lecture*, Eric? Something about walls being there to keep people out when they don't want it bad enough."

Eric shakes his head slightly. He never knows what book I'm talking about.

"I rang the buzzer to be let out. I thought you would be waiting and you'd take me home. When it didn't work, I rang it again. Then I turned around and came back to my room."

I can't tell them what happened next, because they will say it's another delusion, and I will get into more trouble. I can't describe how I was peacefully walking back to my room when they decided to tackle me. I can't remember how many nurses pinned my arms, but for some reason they decided I had to be forcefully restrained while they set up my new room, even though I'd just walked myself back towards them, and away from the exit door, voluntarily. They really don't seem to understand the concept of voluntary and involuntary behaviour here. One of the crazies who apparently no longer required a high surveillance room as much as I did was moved into my room, so I could be moved into his. His needed a lot of cleaning, so they held me while somebody cleaned.

Eric takes a step back from the nurse. He looks from her to me, unsure which one of us to believe. He has never questioned my word before but now, I can see, my credibility is in doubt. The nurse sees an opportunity.

"Sir, we have a lot of patients that need care and we are doing our best for them as well as for your wife. Right now I need to attend to someone else, unless there's something you need?"

She steps away while speaking, before he's had a chance to respond. He stares at me and breathes deeply. I guess I am exactly like the other patients after all. Alone. How will I get out of here?

# 13. Diagnosis

The dark brown man is here again. I never remember his name. I get the feeling he's used to repeating it. I remember his eyes though. They are so green, greener than any I've ever seen in real life, and the whites have been red every time we've talked. Bloodshot. He must work hard.

He stares into me with his piercing eyes that used to scare me. He sits across from me in this small room where people like us go for private conversations. My phoney nurse, Emily, sits to my left. She has not made life easier for me. She looks like a cat: furtive glances, dramatic expressions, and Lisa Loeb glasses. When I ask her a question she gives me a rambling, vague non-answer. Like yesterday, when I insisted that she had changed the clock because I kept losing time. She said she didn't know how to change the clock, which wasn't a precise enough denial. Words are critical, especially to someone who hangs off of each one and takes them all at face value. I think Kitty-cat Emily is lying most of the time, and I can't figure out if it's to protect me or to test me; if she's an enemy or an ally, a caregiver or a warden.

My heart beats too fast. I wonder if they can smell my sweat. I do a casual nose-to-armpit inhale while pretending to flip my hair, to see if I detect any odour. Nobody has offered me deodorant since I arrived and it's something I keep forgetting to ask Eric to bring. Yesterday I asked a nurse for nail polish remover and was pleased that she had some to give me. My chipped nails were getting embarrassing. I feel so much better now that they're clean—so much more presentable.

I realize too late that this man is talking to me. It seems he's been talking to me for a while. Every so often Kitty-cat Emily chips in with her two cents, like it matters, and every so often he pauses and stares at me for a response. Which is what he's doing now.

"Do you understand what I'm saying, Charise?"

I shake my head. I might understand if I'd been listening, but then again maybe not. This is why Eric is supposed to be here. He would understand everything these hospital people are trying to explain. My brain is too tired. I need more sleep.

"Not really," I say.

He starts to ramble again and I try to pay attention. It must be the way he catches my eye and looks at me even more intensely than normal.

"Bipolar Mood Disorder. There are two types, and you are type 1."

"What's the difference?" I ask, not that it matters to me at this point. I just want to respond with something that doesn't sound stupid, to distract myself from the feeling of having been kicked in the gut.

"Type 2 is more mild. People with type 2 have less severe manic episodes, called hypomania. They feel the same euphoria and decreased need for sleep, however there is no psychosis. What you are experiencing is full-blown mania, type 1."

I don't know what he means by psychosis, but I don't want to think about it. I nod, as though his diagnosis makes sense, and in a way it does. Only a few months ago I suggested to my sister that I might be bipolar, because of the euphoria I felt in January after a vacation. We'd come home to a chinook, the strong warm wind that sometimes blows down the Rocky Mountains during winter, creating spring-like conditions for days. Then I'd crashed to feeling joyless and lethargic when winter once again took hold. My sister reassured me that I wasn't bipolar, which made me feel better, but I still knew there was something off. Now, having my fear confirmed as an inpatient doesn't make it any easier to accept. Thinking that I might be crazy and actually being told that I'm crazy by a legit shrink are two entirely different pills to swallow. My throat feels like sandpaper.

Grandy, Mom's Dad, was crazy. He had PTSD from World War II, or as it was called then, "shell shock", was an alcoholic, and experienced sudden and extreme mood swings. Nandy once told me she accompanied him to a hospital while visiting us from South Africa. She saw a sign reading "Psychiatry Department," and she almost died. She almost died because she was married to a crazy person. Good thing she'll never have to know about me. My diagnosis would surely kill her if she wasn't dead already.

"The majority of bipolar 1 patients are diagnosed in their early twenties. A diagnosis at your age is less common."

I almost feel a point of pride. As a lifelong math geek, a petite female robotics engineer, I've always been something of an anomaly.

"Have you been under severe stress lately?" this man asks.

I shake my head. I'm a housewife with a beautiful family, enough money, and not a care in the world. Well, I have many cares, but none of them would be considered *problems* by most of society.

"We need to discuss medication," Dr. Patel brings my thoughts back to the moment.

"Oh, right. You're Dr. Patel," I say. It's reassuring to remember his name while in the grip of insanity. My psychiatrist's name. I guess I have a psychiatrist now.

Dr. Patel starts talking about drugs that I know I won't remember. It's too much. Kitty-cat Emily nods when he pauses, and pretends to take notes. I look at him, then switch to her, then back to him. He is now silent, apparently waiting for a response.

"Okay," I say, with no clue as to what I'm agreeing. He nods. He looks relieved.

"When we first met, you were very paranoid. You kept saying you didn't trust us. Do you trust us now?"

How could I trust them? I barely know them. And everything they're telling me sounds horrible. Where is Eric? I trust Eric.

"Charise, do you still feel paranoid?"

"I'm from South Africa," I say, too quickly. "Of course I'm paranoid."

"Meaning what?" Dr. Patel asks with gentle curiosity.

Growing up in Germiston, a city just outside of Johannesburg, we had broken glass bottle shards embedded at the top of the twelve feet concrete walls separating our properties. We had security bars on every window in our home. We did not play in the streets. We were taught that if we weren't cautious enough we would be car-jacked, raped, or murdered. Racism was instilled in our bones. Paranoia was the key to survival.

"It was part of life. We were all indoctrinated. My mother still unlocks and re-locks the front door five times before she goes to bed, to make sure it's secure. We were taught to fear."

Especially the unknown. Especially strangers. Especially darkness. I don't doubt him because he's brown—only because I don't know him. And he's a psychiatrist, which is scary. And I guess because he's telling me I'm bipolar and can no longer think clearly. I would like to tell him that being born into apartheid and lied to by my government and people I trusted for years has required a long recovery, but I don't think I can explain it right now.

"Charise, while you are in the hospital we can monitor your medications. Once you become an out-patient you will be responsible for it. It's lucky you have such a supportive husband who can monitor you, but ultimately the medications are your responsibility."

I force myself to focus on my breath, just like I do every time one of these people tell me I am ever so lucky to have Eric, because their implication is clearly that a half-wit like me doesn't deserve someone so clever, supportive and charismatic. It's frustrating to hear them praise him so much when they never spare a compliment for me. Sure, he is helping me, and he is great in a crisis, but is being bipolar my fault? Don't I deserve some recognition, instead of being told that I need to be monitored by my husband, and admonished like a misbehaving child? I also don't understand how his support is considered the gold standard. I agree that it's unwavering and I appreciate that, but he's simply doing what needs to get done. Like I would if the roles were reversed. What kind of deadbeat husbands are my medical team comparing him to? And if he's so loving and supportive then where is he now?

I nod. I try to remember what Dr. Patel said before mentioning Eric. I'm not sure what medication he's talking about. Am I on medication? I thought I was just taking sleeping pills because I have so much trouble falling asleep.

"Wait, do you mean the pills I take before bed?"

He nods, staring at me gravely.

"I don't like pills," I say. "Do I have to take them when I can't sleep?"

"Charise, you have to take them every day for the rest of your life."

Somehow this feels like more of a kick than my diagnosis.

"The rest of my life?"

He nods.

"But all I need is sleep. Can't I just take them when I'm short on sleep?"

"No, Charise. The lithium is for your mood disorder, bipolar 1. It's not for sleep, although it might make you groggy." Lithium. They've been giving me lithium? I thought that was a drug from the 1960s.

"But all of this started because I wasn't sleeping. Can't I just sleep better?"

"It's not that simple."

"I have trouble falling asleep. Can't I make it up in the day? Can't I nap?" This makes perfect sense to me. I eat when I'm hungry and use the bathroom when I feel the urge, so why can't I trust my body to tell me when it needs sleep? Any other time when insomnia has been bad I always remember this too shall pass, and it always has.

"No, Charise."

"But why not? Why can't I just sleep when I'm tired? I put a sweater on when I'm cold. Why can't I trust my body to know what it needs?"

There is a comfortable pause while we stare at each other, me waiting for him to respond, and him trying to think of something to say.

"Because society doesn't work that way."

His answer surprises me into silence. What kind of logic is that? Shift workers shift their sleep schedules around all the time. I feel like Dr. Patel is a store clerk telling me he can't process my refund because the computer won't allow it. It's a cop-out. Didn't Winston Churchill take naps all during World War II? And Thomas Edison was famous for sleeping whenever and wherever he needed to. Why was it fine for them, but not for me?

I want to press Dr. Patel more, but I sense the only thing he wants from me is compliance. I will have to wait until Eric comes back. He's allowed to ask questions.

"Your illness is very complicated, Charise. You will likely need lithium for the rest of your life. It is a mood stabilizer."

The word I choose to focus on from that sentence is 'likely.' Likely means possibly not.

"But I'm forty years old and never needed it before."

Kitty-cat Emily makes overly exaggerated eye contact with me as Dr. Patel talks. I avert my gaze. I just want to curl up in the fetal position, right here in this consultation room.

"Where is Eric?" I interrupt. This medical jargon is too much.

They both stare at me, him with compassion and her with a look of annoyance, like, how dare I interrupt the doctor.

"I tried to call him," she says, as though that's a sufficient answer.

"And? Where is he?"

"Charise, we can talk again when Eric is here. I think we should wrap up unless you have any questions?"

I shake my head. Dr. Patel stands, so Kitty-cat follows. Claustrophobia presses in on me and I leap from my chair, mumble a thank-you, and turn around to flee. I yank the door open and rush straight to the nurse's station to ask for the phone. The nurse on duty, Jessica, hands it to me and watches as I start to dial. But after punching in the area code, I have no idea what Eric's phone number is. Is it because I'm bipolar? Do I normally know it? The only phone number I remember right now is that of my first Canadian home, back on Glen Erin Drive.

"Do you want me to dial for you?" Jessica asks.

"Yes, please," I say, handing the phone back across the desk. She finds Eric's number, efficiently punches it in, and passes it back to me.

"It's ringing," she says pleasantly. I step back from the desk and start to pace down the hall. Eric picks up. It sounds like he's smiling.

"I just met with my psychiatrist," I say without a greeting. "And that stupid nurse who hates me."

There is a pause. He doesn't know what to say. He doesn't want me to be angry.

"They told me my diagnosis. Bipolar 1."

"Oh, Reese, I'm sorry." He sounds genuinely sympathetic.

"For what? The diagnosis or because you weren't here?"

Another pause. This time I wait it out.

"For both," he says slowly.

"Where were you? Why weren't you here? They were talking so much and I didn't understand any of it!"

"I wanted to be there—I told them to let me know when the meeting would be so I could be there." Now his voice is starting to rise to match mine.

"Well, you weren't. You weren't here. Where are you anyway?"

I push the button to hang up. Not nearly as dramatic as slamming down a phone but it'll have to do. I miss the olden day phones.

I turn to find Jessica behind me. The look in her eyes says how much she would like to hug me, but they don't do hugs here. I'm not in the mood for a hug anyway. I forcefully extend my arm to hand the phone back before stomping to my room and trying to slam the door, which only swishes softly to a close because of its idiot-proof hinges. This makes me even more infuriated and I want to throw something but there is nothing in here that I can break except for myself, and I'm already broken. I collapse onto my bed, curled into the ball I so desperately craved half an hour ago, and focus on the storm clouds passing by my window.

# 14. Retail Therapy

"Reese, they say you refused your medication last night." Eric is sitting beside me, looking concerned. My cheek is still warm from where he just planted a kiss. He arrived only minutes ago—at first I was so relieved but now I'm sad.

"What?" I sigh. I don't know why they told him that. It's like they just want to keep pitting us against each other. They just want to keep getting me in trouble. I should have signed that stupid form at the start so they wouldn't keep holding it against me.

"The nurse said you refused your medication."

I shake my head to clear it. I try to remember what happened last night—it's all foggy.

"Which nurse?"

"Cat," he says. The name means nothing to me. All of their names are Cat or Katherine or Katrina or Katie or Kitty or Kitty-cat or some stupid thing.

"Last night it wasn't a Cat. It was that older one, she's always muddled."

"Okay. Did you refuse your medication?"

I sigh again.

"I'm getting to that. She came to give it to me when I was doing yoga. I asked if I could try fall asleep without it because maybe I wouldn't need it since my sleep is getting better. I said I would come and ask for it if I couldn't. She said that would be fine."

"But, it was your lithium, Reese. It's not for insomnia."

"Oh. I thought the morning one was my lithium." I don't know. How am I supposed to keep track when they give me so many pills, and each time they want me to check as though I have a clue what the pink ones do and how many white ones I'm supposed to take. "Why did she say it was fine, then? Anyway, I couldn't fall asleep so after a while I went and asked her for the pills."

“So, you took them?”

“Yes! That’s what I’m saying. I never refused, I asked if I could try without and she said it was okay. And then I asked for them anyway. How is that refusing?”

Eric nods.

“Okay, Reese. They didn’t tell me the whole story. I’ll go talk to them.”

I turn back to the window as he walks away. They never tell him the whole story and they never even ask me for mine. They just report me to Eric, then he asks me, and then he has to go back and explain. I don’t understand why there is such a difference of opinion about the same situation. When the people who keep insisting I can trust them use accusatory language—“she refused”, “she tried to escape”—to describe my innocent mistakes, it’s a betrayal. I’m a child whose teacher is reporting bad behaviour to my parents, rather than an adult trying to work through a major diagnosis and a health crisis. I look out the window to see clouds that simultaneously look stormy and calm. They reflect my mood perfectly.

Eric’s voice carries from the hall. He’s doing his charming act, throwing in a laugh every so often, and the nurse’s response sounds appreciative. I hate it. I know he’s putting on this show to help my cause, but it doesn’t feel like that. It feels like they’re in cahoots against me. Plotting together to make the crazy lady feel worse—more alone.

Eric walks back into the room, a big smile on his face.

“Okay, she said we can go for a walk.” No more mention of my refusal to comply, so I suppose he smoothed it over.

“I can leave?” I lean forward from my window seat.

“We can go for a walk through the hospital,” Eric says. He stares deeply into me, as though he’s trying to convey a message. He seems cautious. Or secretive. I don’t know which. Maybe both? Maybe he’s finally busting me out of here? I’m reluctant to get my hopes up again or do anything they'll say is bad, but I remind myself: *trust Eric.* He's the stable one. He doesn't have bipolar 1.

I walk to my closet, which is more of a cubby, and quickly scan the contents. What should I bring? I don't want to leave anything behind if we're not coming back, but I also don't want to be too conspicuous. If Eric's breaking me out then surely he's already thought through how we'll get my stuff. Or maybe he's decided that losing everything is worth the sacrifice for my freedom. I think I need to be coy, play along since he's being so secretive. My heart beats quickly.

"Are we going outside?" I ask.

"Do you want to go outside?" He puts one hand on my back while staring into me with loving eyes. Is this a trick question? Are the nurses listening to see if we're plotting something? I think they rifled through my journal, but did they bug my room too? I better stay safe.

"I just want to know if I should bring my jacket." I stare back at Eric. "Or my sweater. I just want to know what to bring."

"Sure, bring your jacket. Or your sweater. Or both." He rubs my back momentarily before dropping his hand to his side. His response did not make anything more clear. I walk towards the wall cabinet and reach for my sweater on the top shelf, but it's too high, so I step up into the cabinet using the low shelf as a ladder. Then I realize what this looks like. I am literally climbing the walls. I glance back to see if Eric's noticed, but he's turned away to make my bed. I climb back down, put on my sweater, tie my jacket around my waist, zip my wallet into one of the pockets, and put on my running shoes. They're the fastest footwear I have.

We start down the hallway and I make a point of acting nonchalant.

"Can you take a picture of that?" I point to a sign beside the elevators advising people to wash their hands and cover their coughs. It's just the right combination of words and images, and is appealing because of the colours and graphics. I want to hang a copy in the children's bathroom so I can stop having to remind them. I am so tired of nagging.

Eric dutifully pulls out his phone.

"Do you want to be in the picture?" he says.

"No, I just want the sign." I hear the irritation in my voice, so I lean lovingly against his shoulder to force away my mild frustration. Do I still need to explain everything about parenting? That's an old frustration, from before. A normal frustration that every mother I know has at times. I want my old frustrations back instead of what I have now.

We continue to walk through the hospital corridors and Eric patiently snaps pictures of all the signs and art that I ask him to document. Eventually, we make it to a set of doors leading to a courtyard. He doesn't stop me from venturing outside, so maybe his plan is for us to simply walk away from the hospital. Maybe he's parked the truck across the street.

"Do you remember the Mad Genius, Eric?" I ask as we push open the doors. The fresh air and colours attack all of my senses, but I force myself to keep acting casual. I focus on the calming raised garden beds that were planted by patients like me, according to the sign.

"I remember you talking about the Mad Genius." He lowers his voice as we walk past a security guard. Eric nods and the guard nods back; it's as though they have a secret code. Does he need their approval before we can break free? Or is he trying to keep me calm because any disturbance will cause them to pursue us? The guard yawns as he walks through the door that Eric holds open for him. Is that a signal? I watch him continue down the hall but he doesn't look back. I don't know if that's good or bad.

"What about it, Reesie?"

I turn to look at Eric, who is still holding the door open and staring at me.

"What about what?"

"The Mad Genius."

"Oh, right. I wanted to tell you something about that." But now I can't remember what it was. I'll have to wing it so I don't look stupid. "Just that a genius is often mad. So maybe this makes sense."

He looks at me with what seems like a glare but I'm not sure. I can see that he's thinking about something but I have no idea what.

"Maybe," he says after a long silence. He props his elbow out beside his chest for me to take, which I do, and we begin to walk around the gardens. Every so often we pause to admire a flower. I don't know why we haven't left yet but it seems like maybe he's waiting for something. Maybe he needs a final signal.

"I just love these raised beds! We should build some for our vegetable garden," I say, leaning on Eric's chest as he wraps his arms around me.

"Okay," Eric says. After a few minutes, he guides me back into the hospital and points to the lounge area beside the doors. I'm taken aback. Why are we inside again? When is this escape going to happen? When are we going to leave?

"We still have some time left," Eric says. "Do you want to sit?"

What is he talking about? Are the nurses still listening? What is he waiting for?

The same security guard from outside approaches from behind. Surely that can't be a coincidence. Eric glances up at him and they exchange the same knowing nods.

"Is he in on it?" I whisper into Eric's ear. He recoils to look at me, confused.

"In on what?" he whispers back. So they are listening, otherwise why would he whisper?

"Getting me out," I whisper again. "Is he helping? What are we waiting for?"

"Getting you out of what?" This time Eric's voice is not a whisper. He looks confounded.

"Here!" I whisper shout. "I want to go home. I miss the kids."

He stares at me and then his face softens. He pulls me into his chest.

"Reese, we're not going home yet."

I pull away from him.

"What? Wasn't that the whole point of this walk?"

He shakes his head slowly and starts to shush me, which frustrates me even more. Tears well up. I can't believe he led me on like this. Yet another betrayal. So much for *trust Eric.*

"You know, nobody gets mad at the seasons when they change. Maybe if everybody just accepts my moods with love and support rather than fight against them with drugs and confinement I might fare better. Doesn't depression feel like winter to you, Eric? I only learned how to appreciate the cold after we moved to Calgary and I embraced it. My moods are just my seasons. The summer sun is magnificent until it burns too hot when we don't protect ourselves. Especially with someone like me. Sensitive." I don't know where these words come from, but they all tumble out as though rehearsed. I guess it's a theory my subconscious has been working on. I guess it needed to get out. I look to Eric, hoping against hope that my words will reach his mind, his heart. That he'll say the right thing and I can trust him again.

"We have to go up soon, Reesie. Do you want to keep walking?"

I turn and walk away from him. He immediately follows. I want to put my fast running shoes to the test. I'm so angry that I want to run all the way back to my room and slam the unslammable door. But I'm not that crazy. The nurses don't need more ammunition. We walk past people in wheelchairs who look sick—really sick—and my troubles feel small in comparison. So I'll stay locked up in this hospital prison for longer, whatever. More of a break from cooking, cleaning, laundry, and nagging. I stop and turn to face Eric.

"Can you please bring the kids to visit tonight?" Even though I am still furious and disappointed, I force my voice to sound calm. The more rational I present, the more they will all believe that I am. Eric smiles at my suggestion.

"That's a good idea." He puts one arm around my waist. I am still mad at him but I let him leave it there and we start to walk together, step by step. We both slow down to peer into the gift shop window. There are colourful clothes, jewelry, and inspirational quotes carved into wooden blocks. I'm struck with another good idea.

"Can we stop in here?" I ask. Eric checks his phone.

"We have a bit of time."

"Okay. Let's go in and you choose one thing for me and I'll choose one thing for you and then we'll have each other's gift to feel better while we're separated." I don't think Eric understands that this is meant to be comforting, but he'll be home with the kids and his regular life so I also don't think he needs much comforting. I, on the other hand, do. I need a lot.

"Okay," Eric says in the familiar, placating way he agrees to everything that I suggest these days, from raised garden beds to weekly Church sermons.

We walk into the store. My eyes are drawn to a pair of cozy slippers with a picture of a bear and the word CANADA on each. They would better suit a tourist shop than a hospital gift shop, but somehow they make me feel better, as if I'm just on a weird vacation. Soon I'll go back to my normal life. I notice Eric looking at the dressing gowns on a rack outside the store, but I quickly turn my head. I would prefer a surprise. I find the slippers in Eric's size, and stroke them gently. They are softer than they look, and will provide just the right kind of comfort I would like to provide. I hope he'll wear them. I would wear them. Maybe I should get myself a pair. I stand at the counter debating this while waiting for Eric, and after another minute he approaches. In his hands he delicately holds a dark blue silk robe with a large dragon embroidered on the back. My mind starts to spin to try to figure out exactly what message he's trying to convey, because why would he give a recently diagnosed bipolar woman with a dragon obsession something so specific unless there is a reason? I tell my mind to settle down and miraculously it does. Then I reach to hug Eric while he takes out his credit card.

"Thanks," I say. "I love it." I will wear my new robe after he leaves, and it will help me to feel loved. It will shade me from my too bright sun.

We walk back to the ward and Eric signs me in. I put my robe on, we say goodbye, and I'm left alone. I sketch and snack and stretch and then, just when I'm about to go back to the nurse's station to find out what time it is, Eric returns. And he's brought visitors: the kids and my mom. I'm still wearing my robe.

The kids don't like coming here. The patients make them nervous. The staff make them anxious. They don't want to be here. None of us do.

"Give mama a hug," Mom says to the boys and Suzie, who clings tightly to her hand, reluctant to release it and take the three steps towards my outstretched arms. Alex is the first to bridge the gap, so Jack follows. Suzie requires more persuasion before she finally lets go of her Nona and runs into our group hug. They smell so good.

Eric says they've been here before but I don't remember it. Surely not, surely I would remember it. I give them a tour: the exercise bike, the fish that sometimes seems dead, the table with art supplies, the television. The boys want to play video games and Suzie wants to colour, so we hang out in the common area. I make tea for my mom and instant coffee for Eric. The kids are thrilled to be given a juice box from the refrigerator's common shelf. I feel like I'm entertaining and I want to make a good impression. We are all quiet—a combination of tired and uncertain. Before long, other patients start to wander into our space after returning from their off-ward excursions.

"Let's go to my room," I say after making a few introductions. The kids don't want to be on display. There aren't often children on this ward and when there are, they are a sight to behold. Something hopeful.

"Can we go to the library?" Suzie asks.

"Pack up the markers, sweetie," I say. "How do you know about the library?"

"We went last time, remember?" She starts to clean up. We rearrange the colouring pages into a neat pile. A lot of the papers have images of dragons. I pick up the dragon we've been colouring together.

"Should we keep it?" I ask.

Suzie nods. I'm relieved. I never want to throw our art away.

"So, can we go?" she says.

"Yeah, can we?" Jack chimes in. Alex looks over expectantly.

"Not tonight, guys," Eric says. "We have to leave soon. We'll go next time."

Their faces drop.

"What's so great about the library?" I ask. Our local public library has a children's floor and an entire section devoted to play. It is magical. The library in this hospital is bright and full of books and has computers I can use to email under Eric's supervision, but it's nothing like our library at home. And also, how do they even know about this library? Did we go together and I've forgotten?

"They have those mazes and things on the wall," Alex says, gesturing with his hands to help me remember, which it does. He's talking about the small play area with activity centres built into the walls, like the ones we discovered in the checkout lanes of our grocery store upon moving here.

We walk into my room while I consider their request. I think there's a rule against having visitors in my room, but I'm not sure where we're supposed to go. Our family is too much of a distraction in the common area. People are too demanding of our time and attention. We just want to be alone, together.

"But, how do you know about those play things?" I say. I am perplexed. Could I really have forgotten a trip to the library with my children?

"We went last time, remember?" Jack says. The three of them sit on my window seat, watching me on my bed. I would take a picture to admire after they leave, but I don't have my phone.

"No," I say. I stare at them hopelessly. Eric places a chair beside the bed and gestures for my mom to sit down. They have developed a casual symbiosis in the past few days since her arrival. Eric told me they have conversations late into the night after putting the children to bed, sitting outside on our deck. It sounds therapeutic. It sounds like something I would love.

"We went on our way out, Jack," Eric says to the kids. "Mommy wasn't with us."

I am so relieved that I didn't forget. I'd like to jump up and hug him, but I don't have enough energy to stand, let alone jump. I am worn out.

"Oh, right," Alex says.

"So, let's take her there. Can we go?" Suzie often displays a fierce determination that makes me proud.

"Yeah, let's go!" Jack stands, as though this will motivate the adults to change our minds.

"Guys, I already said, not tonight." Eric finally sits down beside me after puttering around my room to collect laundry. "Next time."

Jack sits back down and the three of them hang their heads. Eric's statement reminds us all that our time together will soon come to an end.

"Does anybody want to see my sketchbook?" I ask. If I can keep my audience captive then maybe they'll stay longer. The children's eyes widen and they eagerly nod their heads.

"I didn't know you had a sketchbook," Jack says. "That's cool they gave that to you."

I pick up my journal from the table beside my bed and flip through it with them, taking care to describe each picture and answer their questions. They are full of compliments. Their awe and appreciation inspires me.

"You always were good at art," Mom says, leaning in to admire my drawing of the Northern Lights. We share a smile.

Too soon, it is time for them to go. We hug and say our goodbyes while still in my room, to maintain some privacy. Then we walk down the hall together and I have to hug everybody again, and I don't want to let any of them go. The kids wrap their arms around me and I start to tear up, which won't do because if I cry then they'll cry and I can't make this harder for them. I blink like flapping butterfly wings.

"Have a great night with Daddy and Nona," I say, forcing my voice to sound upbeat and leaning down to their height. "I'll see you tomorrow?"

Everybody takes turns hugging me, the five of them walk out the door, and I am left alone again. A nurse at the desk smiles as I walk past on my way back to my room, but I look away. I sit down on my window seat and stare outside at the gloomy sky. Suzie has left our dragon picture behind, so I pick it up and finger the outline before holding it to my chest. Tomorrow feels very far away.

## 15. Survival Skills

"I like the way you mix things."

I look up from my oatmeal-on-toast. Nolan, a fellow patient/inmate, stands before me.

"I've never seen anyone mix food the way you do." He's looking down at me, but he's smiling, so I know he's sincere. He pulls out a chair and puts his tray on the table. It looks better than mine.

"How'd you get eggs?" I ask.

"I ordered them."

I cock my head to one side and furrow my brow.

"Didn't anyone show you how to order meals?"

"No," I say. "No one showed me how to order meals."

Nolan explains the process, which is similar to hotel room service, and I thank him before reaching for my tea. I blow on it, take a sip, and grimace.

"Too hot?"

"Too bitter." I fumble through the condiments on my tray. Salt and pepper but no sugar. Nolan watches, fork frozen above his plate, as I scoop the jam out of its package and drop it into my mug.

"There's sugar in the drawer," he says.

I did know that. No one told me but I went through the kitchen days ago to find what I needed to make tea. There doesn't seem to be any kind of system here.

"I know, but I don't want to get up. Besides, this adds sweetness and a berry flavour."

He nods, contemplative.

"So, why the oatmeal on toast?"

"Toast was dry. Oatmeal was wet. Texture matters as much as flavour. When something tastes too much of one thing I add the opposite."

"I think most people would use butter for dry toast. Or jam." He smiles.

"Maybe, but I didn't feel like butter or jam." I smile back. I am not most people.

"What would most people use for wet oatmeal?" I ask, genuinely curious.

"The garbage bin," he laughs. Our conversation feels so normal, just two people getting to know each other.

"My husband doesn't like the way I mix food. He thinks it's a sign of my—" I swirl my hand next to my head to avoid saying the word. "He couldn't get over all the teabags in my cup yesterday. He doesn't understand the logic."

"The method to your madness," Nolan says, but not to me. He stares over my shoulder. I turn, but no one is there. Nolan's gone dark. I push out my chair and he speaks again.

"It looks like you and your husband really love each other."

I nod, a bit taken aback.

"That's rare to see. At least in my world." He pushes his chair out as well.

"I think I'll write a poem about it. About you."

I don't know what to say but it doesn't matter. He's already gone. I stand, carry my tray and dishes to the counter, and walk over to the table of art supplies in the common area.

"Hi Charise," a voice says from behind. I turn to discover another patient lying on the couch. He sits up and gestures for me to join him. This guy is just so attractive. What is he doing in the psych ward? I can't remember his name and I've been here for over a week, so we're too far gone for me to ask it now. I tried to be smart and looked on the white board by the nurses' station, but I couldn't find it. My name was there, as well as Nolan's, Leanne's, and Katie's, but there were too many "Confidential" names for me to apply the process of elimination. Maybe he's famous. He looks like he could be in a band. He comes and goes with that guitar case most days, and seems fine—more than fine. Damn, I'm a sucker for a guitar. Good thing I'm married. Good thing Eric has a guitar. Too bad Eric's not here, I'd rather be talking to him especially now that he's become so sweet. Like when we met.

"You were going to tell me the rest of your story about Katie," the handsome guy says. He has a scruffy beard. I don't usually like beards. Maybe his is attractive because he stares so deeply into my eyes, into me. And for a minute, we don't feel so alone.

I join him on the couch.

"Right. So, she was wearing those FM boots, a short skirt, and fishnet nylons. Tons of makeup. Wild curls. And she just signed herself out. She didn't need anybody else's signature." I'd been amazed when I noticed. I am nowhere near being a patient who can sign myself out.

Handsome guy nods. Keeps staring at me, waiting.

"After she left, my husband came to take me for a walk." This hospital thinks I'm a fucking dog. Dropping Eric into the conversation so casually feels awkward but necessary. I don't know if handsome guy knows I'm married, so I just make it clear. He seems to have a good heart. He would respect another person's commitment. He's not desperate.

"And then?" he asks.

"We went to the parking garage to talk," I say. If he asks why, I'll say we were having a cigarette. It's a reasonable excuse and more innocent than what we were actually doing. "And I saw her get into a car nearby. After a while, she got out and this little weasel guy got out, and they both adjusted their clothes and hair and then he handed her something before he got back in his car and drove away. He didn't even wait for her to go back in the building."

"Wow," he says. His eyes are wide. "Do you think it was money?"

Wow, indeed. This guy is so enthralled by my voice, by me, that he wades through the layers and jumps to the pertinent question. I feel special.

"I don't know. I couldn't see." I tell my mouth to downplay the broad smile it wants to display. "It must have been. I saw her with another man the next day."

"So, Katie's a sex worker," he says. "Huh." He doesn't sound surprised.

I glance at the TV that nobody is currently watching, opposite the couch where we sit. It's a documentary about birds called cassowaries. It prompts me to start talking about Australia, New Zealand, and travelling the world. I really want to keep this conversation going. I really want this friend to stay and keep making me feel so charismatic. My mania has subsided significantly in the past week, and I miss these feelings. I don't want to feel like the drugged out zombie I'm becoming.

Out of nowhere, mid-sentence, handsome guy breaks eye contact to look over my shoulder. I turn, to see what has captured his attention, but there is nothing there. He just looked over my shoulder, away from my words, for no apparent reason.

"I'm sorry, I don't mean to talk too much," I say, wounded. His eyes are back on mine in a heartbeat, but the damage is done.

"No, you're not talking too much," he says. I feel like I might start to cry but I know I must not. Another person I thought I could trust who is now caught in a lie. Soon he'll be talking about me and telling secrets behind my back like the rest of the patients and the staff—even my family.

I move to stand and walk away, but he stops me. He insists that he wasn't bored, I wasn't talking too much, he likes our conversation, he wants me to stay. He is so persuasive and I am so easily persuaded. So I stay, and he asks me a question about my new roommate, who has six kids at home, the youngest only three months old. She sleeps most of the time, so there's nothing juicy to discuss. I think she must have post-partum depression and as a mother, I feel for her. Handsome guy asks if I've talked to Trevor again, the homeless guy who is either schizophrenic or an addict or both. On my first night here we were pacing up and down the long hallway, smiling and exchanging a kind word each time our paths crossed. I imagine mine were some of the only kind words he heard here, since he never had visitors and every one else was scared of him, or something. Later that night, I heard him raging in his room, the one that was mine before the nurses switched us to put me in the high observation room after my alleged escape attempt. I shudder, remembering being there. How powerless I was, how frightened.

"No, Trevor left." I didn't see him go. Eric told me he was gone. He left a garbage bag of stuff here, locked in the locker room, which is also the music room where they let us sign out instruments. I guess his garbage bag was probably garbage.

"What's new with Dylan?"

I've been distancing myself from Dylan. He was kind and genuine, but he led me astray in my early days here. When I first rambled about losing time, he remarked that the clocks are funny in here, and this reinforced my theory that the staff were controlling time. He gestured about nurses and patients behind their backs while they were talking to me, trying to convey messages I could only guess at because he never remembered his intentions when I pressed him on them later. Instead of focusing on my recovery, I wasted time obsessing on his hidden meanings, adding them to my list of delusions and conspiracy theories. I can't blame him though, I'm gullible and he's young. And he has his own problems—something about his parents. He won't talk about them.

"Dylan's having problems with Leanne," I say instead of sharing my own experience. Handsome guy knows all about Leanne. She tells everybody the same story: she's an architect who told her boss she was taking a mental health day, and checked herself in here. Most people don't believe her, but I did at first, despite all evidence to the contrary. Gullible me. Leanne can barely draw. She also tells fantastic stories about her children and her boyfriend, which her mother revealed as lies during a visit, laughing while she ridiculed and embarrassed her daughter in front of the rest of us. I don't know what happened with Leanne's children, or if she even has any children, but she does not react well to my children when they visit. She alternates between kindness reeking of desperation, sadness resulting in tears, or a cold shoulder and death stares. We avoid her and leave the ward, a privilege I've been granted because Dr. Patel decided I've earned it. I am allowed daily walks on hospital grounds leashed by Eric's supervision. After my initial outbursts, refusals, and supposed defiance, I've turned into a model inmate. My "team" is happy with my progress. They finally decided to listen to me when I finally decided to shut the hell up.

As if on cue, Leanne appears at the corner where the hallway meets the TV room. She glances at us impassively, and then walks slowly in front of the television, stopping to stretch and purposefully block our view. We don't react. It's about the same as the cassowaries. After she's tired of trying to annoy us, she continues to the kitchen.

It must be breakfast or lunch—I'm still having trouble keeping track without my phone or a clock—because Dylan rounds the opposite corner and walks to the refrigerator before noticing Leanne.

Handsome guy gives me an eyebrow-raise that says either "Uh-oh," or "This should be good," or some combination of the two. I don't want it to be good. I feel bad for Dylan. Leanne acted like his friend after I retreated into self-care, and now she's turned into a total bitch.

Dylan sees her and they share a look before he speaks.

"What did I do?" he says. He sounds sincere, but what do I know? I take everybody's word at face value and that's been one of the things to cause my downfall. I need to stop being so gullible.

"You know what you did," Leanne hisses in a harsh, quiet voice. She knows that a loud voice will call a nurse and get her in trouble. She's wearing a hospital gown since being stripped of her clothes, her dignity, all her possessions, and forced into a high-observation room. I wish one of these "experts" would figure out that those rooms make us worse, not better.

"If you keep this up, I'm going to tell one of the nurses because I didn't do anything," Dylan says, standing his ground. Good for him. We have so few opportunities to stand our ground in here.

"Okay, baby, go tattle. Get Mommy to help you." Leanne's voice is rich with sarcasm. I don't know if she's saying this intentionally to rattle Dylan because she knows he has issues with his mom, or if it's just another one of her cutting remarks. Either way, she hits her target. Dylan's face turns deep red. He looks like he could be a cartoon character with smoke coming out of his ears. He turns and storms away from the kitchen, away from Leanne, away from everyone and everything.

"Morning," Lydia's voice says from behind the couch. I turn to say hello. Handsome guy nods. Lydia is nice. She's in her fifties and she's gentle. She walks straight past the kitchen to the nurse's station and begins a whispered conversation. She's asking for the laptop they let her use, even though none of the rest of us can use laptops on the ward. I think she might be a social worker or some other part of the medical team planted here like a narc, to learn our secrets and report back to our doctors so they have a more accurate picture upon which to decide our fate. If they use surveillance cameras why wouldn't they use other means to invade our privacy and gather information? I haven't asked Dr. Patel about it. He'd chalk it up to my paranoia and keep me here even longer. Anyway, maybe Lydia isn't a social worker or a narc. She cries a lot.

"What's that guy's name again?" Handsome guy points to the kid who just appeared in the kitchen.

"Tommy," I say, which causes the kid, who must technically be an adult, to look over. I wave. "Morning! Did you call her?"

Tommy shakes his head no, forlorn. He hasn't been here long but already he is another one of Eric's adoring fans, and he likes our kids, so he has asked me for relationship advice. He met a young woman at university before cracking from the stress of final exams, and says that they were on the brink of a relationship. Now, since becoming a loony bin inpatient, he fears she will reject him.

"Just call her," I say. "Do it after you eat."

Other people start arriving for whatever meal will soon be served. The woman who had major control issues during gardening therapy, and trashed a public washroom on her way back to the ward while Eric and I overheard from a nearby couch. The angry man who only calms down when he plays the ukulele. The old man who doesn't say anything and can't do anything for himself, and the young one with the devil's fingernails whom I met in the ER. We are a motley crew, that's for sure. Some furious, some elated, some miserable, and some catatonic. All of us trying to get our shit together. All of us human beings. All of us deserving of love and respect.

# 16. My First Night Out

"I'm signing out for dinner," I say to the nurse behind the desk. This is the first time Eric will be taking me off hospital grounds. I don't know the protocol, and I don't want to screw it up. No one explained it to me. Dr. Patel informed me this morning that I'm allowed two hours off-site, but I'm not sure if the nurses know. I've seen people write their initials or the time or maybe both on the white board when coming and going, just like when I go off-ward for a walk around the hospital with Eric, so I'm guessing that's what she'll tell me to do. I feel the need to get permission though. I don't want them to accuse me of being disobedient again.

This nurse is efficient, not friendly. I can't remember her name but I think it's Darlene. She doesn't like chit chat or my questions about lab equipment. She's a decade or so older than me, with dark brown hair from a box. No highlights or lowlights and too much of a grey skunk stripe at her part. Her wire-framed glasses pinch the bridge of her nose in a way that looks uncomfortable. It is either the constant physical tension or merely the dissatisfaction with her life that keeps her face in a permanent scowl. She glances up at me with pressing eyes and a head snap that demands respect.

"I'd like to sign out for dinner, please." I feel my cheeks turn red. "Dr. Patel granted me an offsite pass this morning, so we made plans." Eric stands with my mother and children at the other end of the nursing station. I'm not sure why they're there and I'm here, I guess he thinks I can handle this. Apparently he's giving me too much credit. My family laughs about something and my heart aches to join them. This is the first time I get to leave the hospital for more than a short walk around the building. This is the next step towards my freedom.

Darlene repeats my request and I'm not sure if she's talking to me or to herself. She looks down at her desk and rifles through papers before finding the one she wants. With one pointer finger she scrolls down what looks like a list and then taps three times when she arrives at the point she's about to make.

"It says here that you already used that pass for today." She looks up at me, keeping her finger in place as though she can't lose the spot. I tilt my head. I don't understand.

"No, I was outside with Barbara and everyone, not my family." Barbara runs our group therapy. She is lovely, although I get the feeling that she would like me to talk less.

"The pass is for one hour of technology or two hours off-site and your husband brought your laptop this morning."

I stare at her, dumbfounded. Was that this morning? Is that what the pass dictates? I hear silence from my family and realize that Eric is now beside me.

"Is there a problem?" His voice booms louder than I think he intended it to.

"Yes," Darlene takes over. "Charise used today's pass when she used the computer you brought this morning."

I stare at the floor. Images of us in a restaurant booth surface and slowly start to shimmer, like a desert mirage, until they disappear. The worst part is, what Darlene is saying is vaguely familiar. I think Dr. Patel did explain that I could have one or the other, but not both. Until this moment I had forgotten. I rest my hands on the counter for support. I can't look at Eric, my mom, or the children. I can't show them the tears forming in my eyes, or see their crestfallen faces once again. I am a colossal fuckup.

"That wasn't what we understood," Eric says, aware that I need him to take over. They discuss the miscommunication, her lack of authority, and the specifics of the pass. I watch Darlene's hand reach for the phone as his voice grows louder, and I wonder for a moment if she's calling security to have him removed from the ward.

"The whole family has come to take Charise out for a nice dinner. Isn't there anyone else we can ask who does have the authority to allow it?"

"Well, yes, sir, that's what I was about to suggest. I can phone our on-call doctor to grant an exception if you'll give me a moment." Sir. I've never heard her call anybody 'Sir.' She has the receiver up to her ear. Eric makes a deferential hand gesture that conveys annoyance and appreciation in one fluid motion. Darlene explains the situation to the person on the other end of the line in three succinct sentences. It sounds promising. She hangs up the phone and looks back towards Eric.

"All right. You need to sign out on the board just like you do when you take her off-ward." I wait for her to say something akin to 'have her home by midnight,' but she's not playing games. I stifle my smile in case she thinks I'm mocking her and decides to revoke privileges.

"This will only be for today as you need to discuss with Dr. Patel whether she can have more than one pass for the same day."

Eric is nodding and thanking and shuffling me towards the door as he writes on the board. Mom, Alex, Jack, and Suzie all stare at me hopefully, and their eager, pleading eyes begin to smile as I hug them.

"Let's go," Eric pushes us along before Darlene can change her mind. We walk out together, the six of us, with arms intertwined, feeling like we just got away with something. We hurry to the elevators, through the main floor, and downstairs to the parking garage, and it is only then that Eric and I reach to hold hands, make eye contact, and breathe a shared sigh of relief.

Dinner is nice, but disappointing. Because of my curfew, we have to choose a restaurant close by and there aren't many options. We pick Ricky's All Day Grill, thinking that it will be fun for the kids, but we are wrong. It is dark, grungy, and the food is not appetizing. We all do our best to make lighthearted banter about school, Mom/

Nona driving my minivan, and the rock wall I climbed for group therapy, but I feel a grey cloud hanging over us. It could be because of the impending deadline or the depressing meal, but I think it started to form when I was almost denied access to this night out. When I was almost denied access to something that I used to take for granted: *my* life. What has happened to me that I have to beg permission from a grumpy stranger to share a meal with my family? What has happened to me that these people who were strangers ten days ago now hold so much power over my life? How will I get things back to normal—myself back to normal? The grey cloud fills up with rain as the worst question comes into my mind: what if I never do?

# 17. Friendship Anchors

"Charise, are you awake?" a nurse pushes my door open and walks into my room.

"Yes," I say, perplexed. Shouldn't I be awake? We just had breakfast and the sky is bright outside my window. I don't think I'm supposed to sleep now, but I never know what they want. The rules seem to change depending on who's working, and I can't keep up with them because nobody tells me what they are. I know they want me to sleep—it's critical for my recovery—but do they want me to sleep all the time? I'd like to ask, but at the beginning I asked everything and Eric said to stop, so I stopped.

"Is something wrong?" I say after a beat. I hope this question is okay.

"No, you have a call."

She hands me the phone and I take it even though I think one of the rules is that we can't have the phone in our rooms.

"Hello?" I say into the receiver as I nod my thanks to the nurse, who smiles and walks away. She leaves my door open, so maybe that's sufficient for eavesdropping. Or it's tapped. Who knows? The sign at the front still says "Today is Thursday." It hasn't changed since I arrived twelve days ago. And the fish that swims in the little bowl at the nurse's station often looks like it's dead but the next day it's swimming again, so I'm learning not to take everything at face value here in the psych ward. This is difficult, especially since Dr. Patel and the nurses and Eric and everybody keep telling me that I need to trust them. It is hard to trust when there are so many inconsistencies.

"Hi Charise, it's Annie."

This is a pleasant surprise. Annie is a friend, but not a close one. Our daughters are in preschool together. She moved here from England, so she knows what it's like to be an isolated stay-at-home mom.

Still, we hardly know each other. I am both embarrassed and comforted by her call. Her accent cheers me up.

"Annie! It's great to hear from you," I say, forcing myself to speak slowly. This is my first non-family conversation, so I'd like to come across as relatively sane. "How are you?"

"Good. Same as usual." She talks about her kids a bit. "But, how are you?"

"Oh, fine," I say.

There is a pause, which starts to become awkward.

"I guess you heard?"

"Yes. Ethan's mum told me."

Another preschool parent. So I guess my situation is making headlines around town.

"Have you heard of Stephen Fry?" Annie asks.

"No."

"He's a British actor. He's quite open about being bipolar."

She starts talking about a documentary and I half-listen, on purpose. I don't want to overanalyze, or overreact. It's a shock to hear her say that word: *bipolar*. The word I keep thinking about but don't want to say aloud. Annie said it as calmly as if she had told me this actor is quite open about being bald. Or tall. Or British. At first I'm taken aback, but I quickly realize that the way Annie is talking about it makes me feel more normal, like it's not that big a deal. Everyone else makes it seem like it's the end of the world.

"Thanks, Annie, I'll look him up when I get out of here." Whenever that is. Still no definitive word from my psychiatrist. "What's his name again?"

She spells it out for me, and I write it down. There's no way I'll remember.

"What do you do in the hospital all day?"

Good question. The days pass quicker doing nothing than when I'm busy at home.

"Eric visits with the kids. When they're not here, I draw or write. I've started playing the ukulele. I exercise. I see my doctor. We go for walks. There's group therapy too."

"Is that like sitting in a circle, talking?" Her questions are probing but kind. I like them.

"No. Patients don't know much about each other. We're just in a group doing an activity. We planted a garden, did a drumming circle, had an art class. We did rock climbing one time."

"You did? Where?"

"In the gym downstairs."

Ringing the bell at the top of the rock wall was the most empowering moment I've had since being hospitalized. It was a small group that day, less than ten people, but when they noticed I was near the peak, they started cheering. No pity, jealousy, or sarcasm, only encouragement. It was so motivating.

"Sounds like you won't want to leave." Annie laughs. We both know she's joking, but it makes me sad. When I was first admitted, I joked about how this was a low-budget mom spa. There were a variety of scheduled activities, just like on a cruise, and I didn't have to cook, clean, do laundry, or lift a finger. But the joke quickly wore off. I've been at this spa too long. I just want to be home with my family.

"I texted you a picture of the girls yesterday. Did you get it?"

"Oh, thanks! No, not yet. I'm not allowed my phone in here. I'll check when Eric takes me off ward."

"You're not allowed your phone? Why not?"

"They don't want us on the internet. Don't want us to post anything to social media." I think a nurse told me this. I think someone also said that cell phones interfere with the machines. That seems like an old excuse, but I've had some old nurses. Maybe it's to limit screen time, which worsens insomnia and depression. Or maybe it's so patients don't spend all their life savings online. Or maybe they've caught too many bored, isolated, hypersexual patients masturbating while watching porn.

"That makes sense," Annie says. "Still, it must be difficult."

"It is. I had no idea how much I relied on my phone. Now I have no clock, calendar, music, camera, notes, reminders, email, or internet."

"Yes, I hadn't thought of everything. Sounds like torture."

She's joking again, but her statement rings true. It feels like torture. Our phones are our safety blankets and our final connection with our former selves. It feels like depriving us of them is another way for the medical staff to enforce control. To enforce compliance. To destroy trust. How can I trust someone who takes everything from me and tells me it's in my own best interest? Or doesn't tell me anything at all—just imposes arbitrary rules with no explanations?

I'm tempted to ask about the preschool, teachers, other moms, and other kids, but I have no interest. My brain is too full.

"Well," I say, "I should get going. We're supposed to stick to a time limit on this phone." This is true, although this doesn't seem to be a rule that is enforced.

"Oh, right, that makes sense. Well, I hope you feel better soon."

"Thanks, Annie. Thank you for calling." I feel tears well up, which surprise me. It's not like we're best friends. But still, she called. And listened. And shared relevant information that she thought could help me. She must care. "I really appreciate it."

"Let me know if you'd like me to track down some of Stephen Fry's work. I think you'd like it."

"Thank you. I will." I look down at my notebook where I wrote his name. There are fresh doodles all over the page, which I don't remember drawing. Mostly flowers. Flowers are my favourite thing to doodle. They're safe.

I slide my feet into my flip flops to walk down the hall to return the phone. As I exit my room, I do my standard over-the-shoulder glance to make sure I haven't forgotten anything. I've been trying to teach my children this habit for years as it's always helpful to ensure we don't leave anything behind. The single light above my bed is on, so I reach my hand out towards the light switches located on the wall beside my door. I push a button to turn it off, but the main overhead ones light up. I try again with the middle switch, but that reveals yet another bank of lights near the window. I eagerly click the third and final switch, embarrassed that it is taking me so long to turn off a single light. But this only reveals another overhead light, one positioned above my roommate's empty bed. I'm relieved that she's gone home on a day pass. I don't want to disturb her. And I don't want to look like a fool. Now my room is completely lit up and with three switches controlling more than three lights, I'm at a loss. I slump against the doorframe, staring into my room, pressing buttons at random for too long.

"Are you okay, Charise?"

The voice sounds gentle, but I feel guilty, like they'll say I'm doing something wrong, again. I turn to find Linda, one of the nicest nurses, standing behind me. I feel heat creep into my cheeks. Not only am I insane, but I am also no longer capable of working a light switch. I used to wire robots back in the day. Before I lost my mind.

"I'm trying to turn off my lights, but I can't figure them out," I say. I feel like I'm about to cry. I'm too tired to keep up the model patient act, the one where I feel good but not too good and am perfectly capable of functioning like a normal human being.

"I don't know why they're so complicated," Linda says. She smiles a reassuring smile. She then reaches out to press the same switches that I've been pressing, with basically the same results. The lights seem to have their own agenda, turning on when she presses the button she previously pressed to turn them off, and vice versa. She starts to repeat buttons with increasing intervals, and tests combinations of switches together, clucking her tongue when they still take too long to respond properly. Eventually she figures it out, or she gets lucky, and all of the lights finally go to sleep. The room is dark. It looks cold.

"Phew," Linda says. "We sure like to test you in here, eh?"

She laughs, but I'm not sure she's joking. The thought has crossed my troubled mind many times. Why does the sign at the front desk say "Today is Thursday," every day? Why do I stumble upon candy wrappers strewn about as though to see if we're humble enough to pick up garbage, or, alternatively, whether our willpower is strong enough to resist heading straight for sugar? Why is the fish in the fish bowl sometimes swimming and sometimes dead? Why are the condiments in a drawer one day and a cupboard the next? I don't need tests and trickery to break me down further, I'm broken enough. I need sleep, consistency, compassion, and honesty. I need everything to be real.

"How was your conversation, Charise?"

I look down at the phone, still grasped firmly in my hand. I reach forward to give it to Linda. I'm too tired to take it back to the desk.

"It was so nice," I say. It was so nice. I wish I could crawl back into that phone call and not come out until they tell me I can go home. "Thanks for asking. And for fixing my lights."

She takes the phone, smiles, and continues on her busy way. All of the nurses here are extremely busy, but some of them still remember to be kind. To remind us that we're still capable, and still human beings, even if we are mental patients. To remind us that kindness still exists in a world that will now treat us more harshly than before.

# 18. Back to Reality

"And how are you feeling today, my dear?" Dr. Patel sits across from me in a comfortable armchair. My chair is less comfortable.

"I feel fine," I say slowly as I twirl my hair and fiddle with my earlobe. Sometimes these meetings go well, like when he gives me passes for more freedom, and sometimes they don't, like when he told me my diagnosis. That was not a good day. I hope today will be better.

"You've been enjoying your day passes and home visits?" Dr. Patel's eyes are bloodshot, as usual. He smiles sometimes, which downplays the intensity of his eyes. When he is not smiling, he looks too serious. Angry. But maybe that's just his face. He has been kind to me, and comforting in the strong, silent type way. He definitely bonded with Eric. He jokes and laughs when Eric is at our meetings. I guess Eric puts him at ease.

"Yes." This single word does not come close to describing how much I enjoy my family visits. My children treat me like I'm still mom—still me—especially Suzie. But since day one, Eric has advised me to talk less and act calm, so I'm trying. Besides, I could talk for hours about the stories, crafts, meals, and hugs, and it still wouldn't come close to describing how much I enjoy family time. They're the only thing I hold onto when I'm trying to fall asleep in my lonely hospital bed after I return, in the lonely room I share with another polite, sad, lonely woman. They're the only thing I've got.

"Are you still feeling the symptoms you had when Eric brought you here? Grandiosity? Hypersexuality? Irritability?"

My stomach knots as my doctor sets up what feels like a trap. Yes, I was very interested in sex and sensuality, but I often am and am thankful for it after fifteen years of marriage. And I have big ideas and believe in them—grandiosity—but if I were a man, that would just be called confidence. Yes, I was irritable, but who wouldn't be on so little sleep? Almost every symptom feels like it can be explained away, or assigned an alternate label that would add up to intelligence, drive, and creativity. A woman who has it all, not a crazy person. But I know enough not to argue with my psychiatrist, especially if I want to get out of here.

"I'm sleeping better." This is true. I don't know what sleeping pills I'm on, but whatever it is they're helping. It only takes about an hour to fall asleep and I'm clocking almost seven hours nightly. Oddly, I don't feel any more refreshed. In fact, I feel exhausted.

"Wonderful." He looks deep into my soul. "Are there still coincidences?"

How to answer this question and stay honest? Of course there are, there are always coincidences. Just yesterday evening I was at home rifling through the refrigerator while listening to the radio. I heard the deejay say the time, seven eighteen, and at that exact moment I noticed the digits displaying the temperature of the fridge, seven degrees, and freezer, minus eighteen degrees. Seven eighteen. Right now I'm wondering what the initials on Dr. Patel's mug stand for since they're the same initials as my high school sweetheart. My mind works all the time—isn't that a good thing? It makes me feel special. It makes this doctor, and everyone else, think I'm nuts.

"Not really," I say. I don't want to lie, but I know he doesn't want me to talk about the coincidences. I know I'm not supposed to believe in the coincidences, or "see signs," even though I have my whole life, since long before being diagnosed with bipolar 1. Signs from the universe have always been a trusty guide to steer my intuition. Even Eric, who is so practical and levelheaded and not at all sentimental, follows the signs. He chose our wedding date because it was the same number as the house where he grew up. A good omen.

"Colours? Are they still bright?"

"No, but..." I hesitate. I think some elaboration will make me more credible, but it might be misinterpreted and I'm still not sure if

I can trust him. I don't think I'm putting on an act, but it feels like he might suspect it sometimes, so I should voice a little dissent here and there. I can't always agree and answer his questions with a perfectly choreographed response, telling him what he wants to hear so I can get a pat on the head. I'm not acting, but I am suppressing parts of my personality, the ones that will be deemed the craziest. That makes me sad.

"Yes, but...what?" Dr. Patel doesn't miss a beat.

"Most of the colours here are beige or pastel. So, they're not bright anyway." I don't mention the flowers Eric brought me, which were stunning in both volume and intensity. Or the blue Calgary sky I escape into from my window, which is absolutely breathtaking. These are bright colours that are genuinely bright. None have halos, like the trees did when they first started to glow. There is nothing to fear.

Dr. Patel chuckles.

"Yes, that is true." He skims through my paperwork. "The nurses say you have been behaving."

Don't react. Don't react. Don't react. *Behaving*. Is he trying to push my buttons? I have never misbehaved in my life. I swallow my irritation and give a small nod.

"I think we can try one of two things: an overnight pass. Eric can pick you up this evening, you can sleep at home, and then return tomorrow morning."

I feel my mouth forming a smile and I try to stop it from spreading too far. If I appear too excited or too desperate, I'll be labelled manic. If I come across as indifferent, I'll be labelled depressed. I have to get my response exactly right or he'll change his mind.

"That sounds great," I say.

"The other option I think you might be ready for is discharge. Eric can pick you up today, but he would be in charge of supervising you at all times. You would both return for an appointment with me next week, and then on a regular basis for outpatient care."

My head is bursting and if I could see the colours they would all be brilliant—legitimately. I can't believe what Dr. Patel is saying! But he has always been truthful with me, I think, so I just need to confirm that I haven't misunderstood.

"You mean, I can go home today?"

"Yes, Charise. Do you think you're ready?"

I thought I was ready two weeks ago but they kept telling me I wasn't, and they were right. How should I know?

"Yes," I say firmly, taking a leap of faith. I don't need Eric's voice here telling me to just do what they say. For the first time in two weeks, I want to follow their instructions.

"Okay, I will need to talk with Eric to confirm everything."

Yet another gathering of men to discuss a woman's fate. I have faith that Eric won't screw this up for me though. He better not. Dr. Patel picks up a pen and starts to make notes.

"Between you and Eric, are you confident that you'll take all of your medication?" He asks, looking at me over his glasses.

"Yes," I say, even though the thought of medication sours the good news. It just seems so unnecessary now that I'm back to normal. "Dr. Patel, I'm confident that I'll take all my medication. I plan to take it all," I say. He nods. "But, what if I forget?"

"If you forget, you just take it when you remember," he says. He does not appear perturbed by my question, so that's good.

"But, what if I go to sleep and only remember the next morning. Do I take it in the morning and then again before bed?"

"No, then you just take it that night." He scribbles on his notepad. I wonder what he's writing about me. I hope it's not bad. Another thought occurs, but I think I should squash it down. If I ask too many questions, Dr. Patel might lose confidence in my ability to follow his outpatient rules precisely. But then, I need to know all the rules so I don't break one and end up back here again. Who knows how long I'd be incarcerated a second time? My throat feels hot and my heart is beating fast.

"Dr. Patel, can I ask you something else?"

"Of course, my dear." He puts his pen down and leans back in his chair to look at me.

"What do I do when Eric goes to work?"

"What do you mean?"

"My mom will be with me, but I won't be under Eric's direct supervision. I guess he could work from home, maybe. Should he start working from home?"

He stares at me momentarily before again picking up the pen and returning to his papers.

"I'm going to pretend I didn't hear that," he says. It's hard to tell, because he's looking down, but it seems as though a smile is playing on his lips. What does that mean? Is something funny? Should Eric work from home? Can he not see the flaw in the logic of leaving me in someone's care when that person has to go to work? Is being too honest a symptom of bipolar disorder too?

I drop it. Eric can decide what to do since apparently he's the responsible one. Tonight I'll do story time with the kids, kiss their sweet cheeks goodnight, watch TV with my husband, have a shower and go to sleep in my own bed. In the morning, I will wake up and make breakfast. I will see my children off to school and walk the dog. I will finally be free. Life will be normal again.

# PART TWO: *Treatment*

*June 2017*

# 19. The New Normal

"Are you sure you want to do this?"

I turn from the television to glance at Eric, who stares at me from the end of the couch. It's Sunday night and the kids are asleep. It's been a great first weekend home. We drove to the mountains for Nona to explore. We stopped at Bragg Creek for ice cream. It was perfect—just what the doctor ordered. Along with the mood stabilizers and antipsychotic drugs.

"Do what? I'm just watching TV."

"No," Eric says. "I mean start your job tomorrow. Go back to work."

"Of course." I chuckle at my silly husband. I've been looking for work in Calgary since we moved here two years ago, and he knows that. At the end of April, I interviewed to be an engineering manager at an oil and gas company. They called to offer me the job on the day I was hospitalized. They told Eric they were very impressed by me. The fact that I can have a fresh start now is perfect.

"Reese, you just got out of the hospital."

"A week ago."

"Five days ago."

"Basically a week."

"Anyway," he sighs. "I know you want this. And I'll support you. But are you sure?"

I shake my head and roll my eyes, smiling as I lean over to kiss him on the cheek. I know he means well. He just can't see what I see about my new job—that it's exactly what I need. If I'd started this job, or any job, months ago, I wouldn't have landed myself in the hospital. Nobody would ever have suspected that I have a mental illness. I never would have gone over the edge if I'd had a job to fulfill and challenge me, to occupy my time and my mind. To give me something else to focus on other than the meals and the homework and the house and the dog and the stupid little things that literally drove me crazy.

"Your mom suggested we should just try it and if it doesn't work, you can always quit."

Sounds like my husband and my mom have been talking behind my back, which doesn't feel good.

"So, I just want to tell you that we can always change things if they're not working."

Not working for whom? When I've worked in the past, it's only ever been a problem for Eric, because it forces him to contribute more to the household demands. I think part of him really likes me barefoot in the kitchen. A big part. I furrow my brow.

"Okay. Can we watch now?" I point to the screen. "It's getting late and I want to get a good sleep for my first day tomorrow."

"Sure, good idea." He fusses with the blanket and then nestles in beside me, resting his head on my shoulder. I reach for the remote and try to ignore the seed of doubt in my head that Eric has just watered. Dr. Patel planted it when we told him the news, while I was still hospitalized. He expressed concern that starting a new job might be too stressful. Now I find out that my mom doubts me too. It hurts to learn that no one believes in me anymore.

Katherine highlights cells on her spreadsheet and talks too fast and I'm trying to write it all down but now she's doing a pivot table and I have to look at the screen and it's all too much. When did Excel become so complicated? I used to program scripts incorporating Excel into automated systems. I barely recognize this version.

"Does it make sense?" Katherine asks. She looks at me as though there's only one answer.

"I think so." I stare at the monitor. I can't make eye contact with her because my pounding heart will speed up and explode if I do. And I'll cry. I have never cried at work. I will not start on the third day of my new job.

"Okay, good, let's go assemble the tubes."

I exhale with relief as she turns and stands up from her chair. She rolls it over to her cubicle and picks up a box of parts for tube assembly. I stand up to reach for the box—she's eight and a half months pregnant. I am to replace her while she's on maternity leave, and demonstrate my usefulness over the next year so her boss can create a job for me.

"I'm fine, thanks." She smiles tightly. I want to shout at her to accept help when it's offered, but she's a first-time mom and will resist my advice, like I did my first time. I want to tell her all the useful tidbits I learned over the past decade of pregnancies and babies and children, but I know she won't listen. She probably thinks she knows everything, and is tired of unsolicited advice. What she definitely does know is everything about her job, the one I'm to do in her absence. The one that I still know nothing about after almost a week of training. She's been talking so much, flipping through binders so quickly, and explaining products in such rapid fire that I feel overwhelmed. New jobs always take time to learn, I remind myself, but I've never started a new job while taking heavy drugs. They make me feel waterlogged, like I'm swimming through her words and I can't reach the surface.

"Are you coming, Charise?" Katherine calls from the doorway. I nod and quickly turn to follow her, eyeing the kitchen on my way to the boardroom. I've never worked anywhere that provided free granola bars, chips, cookies, and fruit. I wish I'd been faster so I could grab something on the way, but she's already annoyed that I'm lagging behind so I don't think I have time.

She closes the door behind me. Ashley, a technician, is ready, wearing latex gloves and a plastic cap over her hair. She looks like she just stepped out of an episode of *Laverne and Shirley* and I want to laugh but then Katherine hands me my cap and gloves. I put them on, slightly embarrassed about my appearance, but it's just the three of us in this room and we all look ridiculous.

Katherine starts to demonstrate. It looks easy. We have to slip one set of connectors on one end of a pair of tubes, run our hands to the opposite end, and then match a different set of connectors. Everything is colour-coordinated and idiot-proof. The only margin for error lies in the potential for twisting the tubes when we run our hands along them.

"In all the years I've been making these, I've never once gotten the tubes crossed," Katherine says. She smiles at me. I guess she can tell I'm nervous. I wonder if she knows why? I don't know what Eric said about why I couldn't talk on the day she called to offer me the job, right before he took me to the emergency room. I hope she doesn't know that I'm bipolar. I want to be treated normally. I don't want to scare anyone.

We start to build and it goes well at first. I take things slowly and force myself to focus. The work isn't difficult, but it's tedious. Still, I prefer it over trying to understand Katherine's pivot table.

"This one is wrong. The connectors are switched," Katherine says sternly. She looks to me, and I look to Ashley, who is also looking at me.

"Sorry, was it mine?" I ask. Ashley and I are performing the same job and Katherine is doing Quality Control. I don't know how she can tell whose is whose once it's placed in the pile.

"Did the Y-connector have tape on it?" Ashley asks, turning to Katherine.

"No," Katherine shakes her head. Ashley turns to me.

"I've been putting tape on each of my connectors for verification."

Verification for what? To verify that she's perfect and I'm the fuck up? So she can throw me under the bus? Thanks a lot, Ashley.

"Okay, sorry," I say. "I'll pay more attention." But I don't see how I can pay more attention when I'm already doing my best. We keep working. I'm desperate to find the balance between hyper vigilant focusing and not taking too long.

"There's another one," Katherine says and then sighs. "Charise, do you want me to explain it again?"

I tell her no, she doesn't need to, and look down at the connectors. What more is there to explain? My four year-old could do this job. I apologize again and continue working. It's not long before I've messed up another one, and another one, and a few more after that. Despite my best efforts, I just can't get the hang of this stupid menial task. Ashley and Katherine both seem perplexed, slightly sorry for me, and annoyed because I am making us take too long. Katherine has a worried look on her face, which I interpret as apprehension, because if I don't understand the spreadsheets and I can't do basic kit assembly, what will I be able to do after she's gone?

We finish the job slowly. At some point I think I start to get it and I'm not making so many mistakes, but the damage has been done. There is a collective sigh of relief when the last tube is packed away and we can remove our gloves and hairnets and open the door to this airless, windowless room. I am the first to escape, this time without offering to carry the box for Katherine. We both need our space.

I can't do this. Katherine has been training me for three weeks now and I'm no better off than on day one. She will be back from lunch soon and she's expecting this spreadsheet to be finished and I don't understand the first step. I prop my elbows on my desk, rest my head in my hands, and start massaging my temples while trying to decipher the blurry numbers on my monitor.

"Everything okay?" Ashley calls out from her cubicle behind me. I turn to read the look on her face. She doesn't appear concerned, but she doesn't appear pleased either, which is what I have come to expect from Ashley. She is happiest when I am making mistakes. Since the tubing incident there have been a few other times where her motives seemed questionable. I think she wanted my job. I think she wants me to fail. Plus, she's one of those moms of an only child who raves about her daughter likes she's the most precious little thing. Why do parents of only children bother bragging to a mom of three? Clearly I've been there, done that, and had two more opportunities to do it better, so what could Ashley possibly be thinking when she tries to school me at child-rearing? Her only child is not even as old as my youngest. Sometimes it's a struggle not to roll my eyes. At least her condescending faux-concern has disrupted my panic attack that was gearing up.

"Fine, thanks," I say with a fake smile. I turn back to my monitor, my heart pounding.

"Well, I'm here if you need me," Ashley says. This time I don't respond. I'm not interested in playing her mind games. Plus, I'm too engrossed in this cell's formula. I can feel the variables coming together and it's close to making sense when I lean in too much and suddenly, it's all a blur. I move back, then forward, but it refuses to come into focus.

I take a deep breath, try to slow down my racing pulse. Now I can feel sweat on my back, which only happens when I'm truly stressed. When I'm truly about to panic. I slump in my chair and look up at the ceiling tiles. They have no answers for me. I sit upright again, breathe through my mouth, and glance around the office at my coworkers who are all intently focused on their own monitors. Most of them wear looks of concentration, a few are scowling, and one has a big smile on his face. I watch as my diagonal neighbour pushes his chair out to stand up, reaches for his vape pen, and walks toward the office's front door. That simple act makes my heart still for a moment, and then makes it ache. That's what I need: a break. Not a vape pen, that was a failure in Edmonton and I'm avoiding anything that Dr.

Patel would classify as risky behaviour, just a break. I need to get out of this office.

As soon as this realization hits it occurs to me that it's not a break I need. I just need out. I need to quit. I don't need this job. I haven't worked in two years and we've been fine financially. Our family prefers it when I'm not working—I'm there to cook and clean, take care of the kids and the homework and the piano lessons and whatever else needs to be taken care of. That's my true full time job. When I'm working outside our home, everybody else has more responsibilities. Mostly Eric, but the kids too. It hasn't hit them yet this time because my mom is still staying with us, but as soon as she leaves everybody will realize that me working isn't sustainable. Eric was right. Mom said I could still feel good that I tried, even if it didn't work out. I can live with that.

My heart is still beating quickly, but now it's more from excitement than panic. Faced with the awareness that I can leave—that I should quit—it's simply a matter of standing up and walking out the door. And I'll never have to come back again.

Eager to get out, I pack my things as discreetly as I can. I don't want Ashley to start asking questions. It doesn't take long: I've only been here three weeks. I zip up my bag, close the stupid Excel file, and log out of my computer for the last time. I stand up and turn to Ashley.

"I'm not feeling well," I say. She gives me a look I can't read. Maybe concern. "I'm going to go home."

"Okay," Ashley says. "Can I do anything?"

"No, thanks." I smile sweetly and say goodbye. I will not miss Ashley. Or Katherine. Or anybody in this office. Although I will feel guilty when I have to tell my boss. He's gentle. Maybe I should explain about the drugs I'm taking and how they make me slower and more confused. Maybe I could be accommodated with more time until I get used to things. But no, it's too late for that. I've already packed my bag.

I walk to the lobby and as I push the door outwards and step into fresh air and freedom, I realize that I still have the key fob for the front door on my keychain. I'll have to mail it back. I'm not going in there ever again. Eric's been driving me here and Mom's been picking me up, so I don't have a getaway vehicle. That's okay, I'll just walk. It's a lovely day and my heart could use the exercise. It needs to calm down. An eight kilometre walk will be just right.

# 20. Road Trip

"You okay, Reesie?" Eric asks. He turns his head towards me and then looks back at the road. I quietly inhale and exhale, deeply. I know he's concerned, but he asks the same question every half hour and I've already answered it more than a dozen times today. Each time with the same answer.

"Yup," I say. He keeps driving. No acknowledgement, no further investigation. How does he know I'd admit if I'm not okay? How am I supposed to know if I'm okay?

I slide my feet out of their Birkenstocks and prop them up on the dashboard above the glove compartment. My dress slips down between my thighs and I pull it up, smoothing it straight over my knees. I don't want to let myself be too exposed. I don't know what might be construed as hypersexual and used against me at a later time, especially since Eric is being so vigilant right now. Every night before bed he asks me if I took my medicine. I wouldn't mind it if he brought me a glass of water and my pills, so it felt like an act of kindness rather than him policing me. All day he asks if I'm okay, if I'm tired, if I want tea. None of his questions begin an actual conversation. None of them make me feel any better.

"Are you looking forward to camping tonight?" he says.

"Yeah," I say and nod slowly, staring out my window. We left Calgary a week ago and made our way south through Montana, Utah, Nevada, and into sunny California. Highlights of this summer vacation have included an Old Geyser eruption, the Las Vegas strip, the San Diego Zoo, the Santa Monica Pier, and all the nature we've seen everywhere in between. It's been a week of hotels and I am itching to sleep under the stars. Today we're driving to Limekiln State Park, where we'll camp for the night. Tomorrow it's San Francisco. Eric planned this entire vacation. I imagine it took a lot of work. I can't keep track of the daily plan, let alone the two-week plan. My arms feel so heavy that I can barely lift them and my fingers are too uncoordinated to hold a book, not that that matters since my mind is too fuzzy to read a sentence, let alone a novel.

I turn to see what the children are doing. Each one holds an iPad, zombie-like. Of course, because I'm the only parent to enforce screen time limits, and I don't have it in me right now. I look at Eric, who smiles at me as though everything is fine. As though everything is great.

"Man, that traffic was crazy! I think we're through the worst of it," Eric says.

I immediately tense up, but he doesn't notice. I never realized before just how often Eric and the rest of the world refer to bad or bizarre things as 'crazy' or 'insane,' a lazy alternative to a more precise word. I used to do it too, all the time. It irritates me now, but I have been told that I'm too sensitive by all the meaningful people in my life, for as far back as I can remember. So I don't say anything. Maybe I'm too sensitive.

"We're about forty minutes from the campsite," he says.

This also makes me tense. As long as we're in the car, I don't have to do anything. I don't even have to pretend. But the minute we get out, no matter where we are, I am required to act like a normal human being, capable of normal functioning. All I want to do is sit, lie down, or go to sleep. I can't remember the last time I felt this numb. I don't want to be manic again, because the euphoria was not worth the paranoia, but I would like to feel alive. Eric says it seems like I'm swimming just below the water's surface and it takes everything I've got not to drown. I couldn't have put it better myself. I couldn't have strung together any other combination of words to put it better myself. I, a writer, couldn't formulate a coherent sentence in a reasonable amount of time to save my life. Who have I become?

No more mania means I'm not confident anymore. I don't know what to think about reincarnation or religion or art. When I believed in myself, I was able to do anything. I was rapping in the emergency room and it sounded good. At least, I thought it did, and that's all that matters. I miss feeling confident, even if my abilities were all in my head. Now I have nothing but doubt, which means I can't do anything. I don't think my dreams will come true, so there is no point dreaming them. I tell myself this too shall pass, but it still feels hopeless.

Sleeping under the stars was magical. It took too long to pack up our site and get back on the road this morning, which is likely my fault because the only thing I did to help was wash the dishes while Alex helped Eric with the tent. I don't think Eric was thrilled. He's been irritated and twitchy behind the wheel all morning.

He lets out a strange noise: half-moan, half-sigh. It's his sign that he's too tired to drive. It's his way of asking me to take over. I ignore it. Half an hour of silence and intermittent moan-sighs passes before his head starts to drop down to his chest. He catches it each time, only a second after it's fallen, but the message is clear. If I don't take over he is going to fall asleep and we will crash. I don't know if he does these things intentionally for me to offer, instead of asking and admitting that he needs help, but it's become part of our unspoken language. I always offered before the hospital. Now I'm dead weight.

The first time I drove my minivan after the hospital I felt heart palpitations and had to meditate to calm down before I could back out of the garage. I still haven't driven the kids without another adult present. I did a long driving stint at the start of this trip and it wore me out. I can't remember where we started or ended up, but I remember my tight grip on the steering wheel. I tuned out the kids' requests for snacks, movies, and everything else, which I never do, and focused on the road. I couldn't look more than two car lengths ahead of me, for fear that I would crash. Eric fell asleep, the kids stopped asking, and I kept going. When he woke up, I was done. I pulled off and we traded seats. Eric was refreshed and appreciative of how far

I'd driven. I needed to zone out and not be the person responsible for keeping my family alive. I haven't offered to take the wheel since.

"Do you think you could drive, Reese?" Eric says. He must really be exhausted if he's asking. He loves to drive and he hates to be a passenger. He especially hates to be my passenger because I'm too slow and careful.

"Okay," I say, palms already clammy. I have to do it since I've barely done any driving during this trip and he's about to fall asleep. He would too. Unlike me, Eric can fall asleep anytime, anywhere.

He exits and pulls to the side for us to switch. I climb over the console between our seats while he walks around the front. He reclines his seat as soon as he's back in the car, before he puts on his seatbelt. I punch our destination into the GPS. Eric watches me and begins to explain the route, how simple it is, and what exit to take. He doesn't seem to understand how jumbled my mind is. There is no way I can pay attention to exit signs while trying to keep our family safe. I nod to placate him, but say nothing as I pull back onto the road. I think the words "Please, God," and my sincerity surprises me. If I were religious I would pray. But I'm not religious. I'm nervous and terrified. And bipolar.

I watch the minutes on the clock as we approach our destination. I stay in the right lane except to pass, and each time I move into the passing lane it makes my heart race. I can't drive too close behind the slow cars though, so it has to be done. Driving too close behind any car also makes my heart race, as does driving alongside an on-ramp full of cars that want to merge into my lane. The minutes tick by slowly. I have no idea what scenery we pass. Eric sleeps, the kids stay on their screens, and I watch the clock and the road. After almost two hours the GPS tells me to exit and I release a breath I hadn't realized I'd been holding. I pull off of the highway and do as I'm told: right, left, another left, arrived. I pull into a parking spot and turn off the car, which makes Eric wake up.

"Oh, great, we're here," he says, his voice gravelly.

Yes, I think, we made it somehow. I know this should feel like a win for me, that getting us to our destination safe and sound should feel like an accomplishment, but it doesn't. It feels like a little thing that other people do without a second thought or a pat on the back. It feels like one more thing I can't do well, and won't do well again. It feels bittersweet. I hope Eric doesn't ask me to drive ever again.

# 21. Telling People

September can be stormy in Calgary, but this particular Friday morning is gorgeous. Sunshine and blue skies surround us, and it is mild and balmy. It's the end of the first week of school, and we've almost made it to the weekend. I feel apprehensive walking Alex from our house to his bus stop, even though we've done it together for four days in a row. I'm never certain who I might run into during school dropoff.

It's been four months since my manic episode and diagnosis. At first, I didn't hesitate to put it out in the open. We told good friends, who looked after our children and dog, and delivered meals during the initial difficult time. I didn't realize how many good friends I had made here. I told Eric to speak freely about it with his work colleagues, which he did. I did not feel ashamed about being bipolar, so there was nothing to hide. My miscarriage years ago taught me to speak up about hardships, even the ones that have a stigma, so talking about being bipolar feels like an extension of that. I often remind myself of a Dr. Seuss quote, "those who mind don't matter, and those who matter don't mind." Since May, I've shared my story on social media, my personal blog,and an inspiring and supportive website called Option B, created by Sheryl Sandberg to help people build resilience in the face of adversity, as a way to help others. It's been cathartic to write about my mental health, and the feedback I receive encourages me to continue. It replaces isolation with connection.

But this week, the first week of September, my safety bubble has burst. I'm out in the open, walking my kids to and from school. I'm seeing moms I know but don't know well. I'm interacting with teachers and hockey parents. People I am friends with online but not really in real life. Acquaintances. I don't know what they know about me, how they feel, or how I'm coming across. I can't tell if they're just being nice, or if they would schedule playdates at which I would be in charge of their children. Do they fear I'm violent? How will school staff react if my children talk about my hospitalization or how I made them a dinner out of compost? How I have a psychiatrist? Will somebody report me if I yell on the playground? Jack often takes risks on the monkey bars that scare me. It's almost like I need a stage director instructing me on how to behave so the scene doesn't fall apart.

I see three adults lingering around the bus stop as Alex and I approach. It's the same two dads who have been here all week: Kevin, a neighbour and friend who has been quietly supportive in an I-don't-know-what-to-say-but-I'm-here-for-you way, and another man I barely know who seems nice. I can't imagine that our neighbourhood grapevine has prioritized my mental health status enough for him to know, but even if he does, he doesn't seem like the type to care. Alongside them stands another woman I recognize who hasn't been doing the bus stop drop off this week. I know her, but not well. Her name is Kate. We met last year through a local moms' group, and have had a handful of conversations at the events. We're Facebook friends, and she's commented on some of my posts so she knows I'm bipolar. My heart speeds up as my feet slow down.

"There's the bus," Alex says as it turns the corner onto our street. We're almost at the stop, so we don't need to run.

I focus on Alex. He's eleven years old and in grade six now, so I know not to hug him anymore, as much I would love to lean in and hold him close. He says a quick goodbye and climbs the stairs into the bus. I watch as he chooses a seat near the back and gets himself settled. I watch because I want to see him for as long as I can, but also to avoid conversing with the adults.

After a few minutes, the bus closes its door and pulls away. I don't wave, even though I want to.

"And they're off!" A voice says behind me. I take a deep breath, force a smile, and turn to face the three of them.

"TGIF," I say slowly, to be sure I sound calm. Kate is struggling with her dog's leash because her dog and Kevin's dog want to wrestle. I watch them momentarily and realize too late that I should have taken the opportunity to leave. It is only after she has pulled her dog free and turned to me that I remember we live in the same direction. I look at Kevin. We all live in the same direction.

"I'm going to give Pepper a long one today," Kevin says. Sometimes these healthy, active Calgarians make me feel so lazy. All I want to do is climb back into bed, and he's squeezing in an energetic dog walk before work.

Kevin waves and turns to walk with the other man, whose name I can't remember. He too has a frisky dog at his side trying to escape her leash. I am the only person who refuses to walk our dog to the bus stop, to avoid this shitshow. And I'm the crazy one.

"Shall we go?" Kate says. I'm filled with anxiety. We fall into stride together, which is not easy because she is a head taller than me, and she starts to talk about school and how her son is adapting. Based on my experience, it is far too early to say. Still, I'm thankful for this casual conversation that has taken us to the intersection where we'll part ways. I'm just about to lift my hand to wave farewell when Kate nods her head forward.

"I'll keep walking with you. Riley could use it," Kate says. She reaches down to rub her dog's side. Her dog promptly lies down as though to protest the extra exercise. I wonder if I can somehow just keep walking while her dog takes a nap. Kate is nice enough but we don't have much in common. I don't like struggling to make conversation, especially now when I have something I could be judged on.

"You know, I wanted to tell you, I read some of your posts through the summer." She stands over her dog as though we've arrived somewhere. I guess we're not crossing the road.

"Yeah?" I avoid eye contact by staring at Riley. I want to trade places with him and just lie down on the sidewalk. As though he read my mind, Riley stands and begins to half-lurch, half-walk again.

"I was wondering, how did you know there was a real problem?"

This is interesting. I've received messages complimenting me for my bravery and thanking me for trying to help the stigma, but not many people have had specific questions. Aside from Dr. Patel.

"Well, in hindsight, the lack of sleep was the first indication. But since that was typical for me I ignored it. When I served my family garbage for dinner, I couldn't ignore that."

"Oh, we've all served garbage for dinner." She waves a dismissive hand.

"No," I say. I don't think she gets it. "Like, actual garbage. From the compost."

Kate turns to me with an unnatural smile and then gives an awkward laugh.

"I worry about my husband. He doesn't get enough sleep," she says.

Not exactly the same thing, but we start a short conversation about sleep habits and how to improve sleep quality. I'm an expert now.

We're almost at my house. If I cross the street diagonally I can say goodbye and walk to the curb now.

"Well, this is me," I say as I step off the sidewalk and onto the grass.

"You know, I just want you to know, everybody's got their thing."

I'm not sure how to take this. Is it supposed to reassure me that it's okay that I'm crazy because other people have issues too? Like, I should just get over it? I think she means well, but I feel like she's downplaying what I've been through. What I'm going through. I guess it's better to have people downplay than overreact. I guess.

## 22. Life Goes On

Shortly before his suicide, Van Gogh wrote, "How difficult it is to resume one's ordinary life without being absolutely too demoralized by the certainty of unhappiness." This is the perfect description of how I've felt lately, of what it's like to go from manic to medicated. Reading books by or about people with bipolar helps me to keep my chin up and feel a sense of belonging to a club. Not a club I would have chosen, but one which is nonetheless filled with talented, inspiring people: Ernest Hemingway, Kurt Cobain, Dolores O'Riordan, Ted Turner, Glenn Gould, Ada Lovelace, Robert Munsch, Jackson Pollock, Lou Reed, Amy Winehouse, Virginia Woolf, Winston Churchill, Vincent Van Gogh, and more. I understand their torment, and admire their contributions to the world. I am sobered by how many of their lives ended by suicide, drugs, and alcohol. I don't want to add to that statistic.

I close *Van Gogh's Ear* and place it on the stack of library books beside my chair. I glance at each spine to decide what to read next, looking for something lighter, less agonizing. I'm glad I found these books but they are an emotional rollercoaster. Before Van Gogh, I read about Suzy Favor Hamilton, an Olympic athlete whose bipolar switch turned on when she became bored in her comfortable suburban life. She moved away from her husband and daughter and became an escort in Las Vegas. So far, my hypersexuality has only been played out on my husband, but what if one day it's not? Before that, I read a book called *Madness*, about Marya Hornbacher's descent and eventual bipolar diagnosis after decades of eating disorders and misdiagnoses. It made me feel both comforted by the shared experience and fearful of the possibilities. Although I'm reluctant to get up from under this cozy blanket, I decide not to read anymore today.

I throw the covers aside and stand up quickly. This startles our dog Piper, who was sleeping comfortably between my chair and the fireplace, and she jumps towards me and leans in to be patted. I oblige her. We're close to the glass patio doors and I look at the snow covering our backyard. The blue sky and constant sunshine in Calgary is wonderful, but also deceptive when it's January and there's two feet of snow on the ground. I take a deep breath and remind myself that this time next week we will be in Mexico for a week of sun, sand, and pampering. I need an escape from winter every year otherwise my Seasonal Affectiveness Disorder sets in. Or maybe it's just the depression part of being bipolar and has nothing to do with SAD. I decide to start packing but I only have enough energy to pull the suitcases out of storage.

Mid-morning I'm supposed to work out but I don't feel like it. It's hard to get motivated these days. All I want to do is sit on the couch and watch something uplifting like *Kevin Probably Saves the World*, or something distracting like *Fargo*. TV passes the time so I don't have to think these sad, lonely thoughts, but they always return at the end of the show.

My phone rings, calling me out of my reverie. Eric's name appears on the screen.

"Hi," I say.

"Hey, Reese. How are you?"

We chit chat while I wait for him to get to the point. Eric rarely calls without a reason.

"How did you sleep last night?" he finally asks.

"Fine," I say. It was the same answer I gave when he asked me before leaving for work this morning. And it's true. I got seven hours of sleep last night. No sleeping pills, no tossing or turning, just lights out and deep breathing. Dr. Patel would be pleased.

"That's good," he says, still beating around the bush. "What are you doing today?"

I pause. I have literally nothing planned.

"I was going to work out."

"Oh, that's great," he says, a little too eager.

"Why is that great?" I ask. I'm legitimately trying to understand his reasoning. I know why it's great, but I'm not sure Eric does.

"Oh, you know, just, to keep your spirits up."

Huh. I guess he does know why my workouts are important. Sometimes he surprises me.

"I thought you were going to tell me to lose weight," I say.

Silence.

"Well," he says. "Can I tell you something? But I don't want you to take offence or feel self-conscious about it."

How the hell do I answer such a loaded question?

"Okay," I say slowly. "But, I'm not promising."

He laughs. He thinks I'm joking. Sometimes he doesn't surprise me.

"It's just that I've noticed you have gained a little weight. I can feel it when I hug you."

I stiffen, but since he's on the phone he can't tell. I guess he hears it in my silence though, because he tries to be reassuring. Tries to take it back.

"And I want you to know that I love the fuller you. I just love your shape."

Okay, that's something. I already know I've gained weight, and the doctor told me to expect this side effect from the drugs. Eric continues on about how beautiful I am and how much he loves me and it sounds like he's trying to placate me. Eventually he reaches the end of a long list of compliments.

"Did you wake up in the night?" he asks.

"No." I want to add that it's because of my late-night snack, like a baby's dream feed, but I don't want to talk about my weight again.

"I guess your snack is preventing the night wakings, then."

Sometimes Eric can read my mind. Last week, he noticed me snacking before bed. It was an unusual new habit. I explained that lithium is easier on the stomach if I take it with food. It also helps me to sleep through the night, which is fantastic. The only thing worse than having trouble falling asleep at the start of the night is having trouble falling back asleep at 4am, when my mind is rested enough to put up more of a fight. I'm impressed that Eric remembers this conversation, and my explanations. He doesn't always pay attention.

"Yes, I think it is." I smile to myself, pleased for his small pat on my head.

"Just, maybe, you might want to cut back on the bread."

My smile is replaced with a strong urge to throw the phone across the room. I can picture it hitting the fireplace mantel and shattering into a million sharp little pieces.

"But you just said you love my shape," I say. My voice is cold, but he laughs as though I'm joking, again.

"Yes, I do, I do. You're right, eat whatever you want."

This is one of the things my husband does very well. Steps in it and then tries to make amends to whomever he's offended using words that are now meaningless.

"I better go," I say. This yo-yoing conversation has tired me out.

"Okay, have a good day. I love you."

So you keep telling me, I think to myself. I hang up without saying goodbye. As I place my phone upside down on the kitchen countertop, my gaze falls upon the suitcases lining the hall. It feels like they're mocking me. I am eager for our winter getaway, but I am also apprehensive. I don't know if I'll sleep well and I doubt I will exercise or eat properly—all factors that could result in mania. But that's not why the luggage mocks me. I don't know if my bathing suit will fit. Up until this conversation with Eric I hadn't considered that possibility. Now it's all I can think about. I know I'm not supposed to read too much into everything, but this feels bigger than just my bathing suit. If it doesn't fit, does anything? Do I fit in my family? Do I fit in my life?

# 23. Outpatient Paranoia

The wind is brisk today, so I pull my hood up and huddle into my coat. The end of February means spring is in the foreseeable future, but we're not as close here in Calgary as we would be in Toronto. Still, I would never have found free parking anywhere near a Toronto hospital, and this stunning blue sky and bright sunshine is a rarity in Toronto's grey, dreary winter. Calgary is freezing, but spectacular. It must make working in a hospital so much better when you can look out the window and see blue sky and mountains even on a bitterly cold day. I don't remember if it helped me as an inpatient and I hope not to find out.

I walk through the revolving doors and a blast of heat hits me. I shake my hood off and stomp my boots.

"Good morning," a voice says, startling me so much that I jump. I've been coming for outpatient appointments with Dr. Patel for nine months but I'm always a little on edge. Today I feel fine, and relieved that our vacation a few weeks ago did not result in mania, hypomania, depression, or anything. Even my bathing suit cooperated. But still, these appointments are high-stakes. What if he deems me manic and admits me to the psych ward based on my behaviour during one visit? Can that even happen? I don't know, and it's not a question I can ask because he might interpret it as anxiety or paranoia. More of a reason to lock me up. Last May I was curious about everything, and Eric kept telling me to stop asking questions. So today, and every appointment, I try to keep that in mind. I try to appear less interested, more normal.

"Good morning," I say to the elderly man in the red volunteer vest standing in front of me. My smile is perfectly measured. It's not fake, but it's not entirely natural either. Should Dr. Patel question my sanity today, I don't know how much he would investigate before having me committed. I must appear normal in case this interaction is recorded by security cameras. I'm conscious of creating evidence to protect myself. I picture being dragged away from Dr. Patel's office kicking and screaming if I don't appear well. Or if I appear too well. I'm afraid that any sign of irritability, frustration, enthusiastic talking, or creativity will work against me, even though everybody feels those things at times. I know I'm not everybody. I have to hold myself to a higher standard. I have to fake it until I make it.

I know my way to Dr. Patel's office. I walk past the café where Eric bought me an overpriced muffin on one of my first off-ward passes, towards the gift shop where we bought each other presents nine months ago. He does not wear his slippers and I have not worn the silk dragon robe since being released from the hospital. I love it, but there is something about it that feels off. Sinister.

I pick up my pace to avoid having to face more memories and to make sure I'm not late. Healthy people can be late without severe consequence, but if I'm late anything could happen. Lateness is a sign of disrespect, which I don't want Dr. Patel to feel. I need him on my side.

I hand over my health card to check in at the Addiction and Mental Health Adult Outpatient Clinic, and then take a seat in the waiting room. It's not long before Dr. Patel calls my name and leads me to his office. He is usually punctual.

"Did a patient draw that?" I ask, pointing at a picture behind where Dr. Patel sits at his desk, and immediately forgetting that I'm not supposed to pose questions or make side conversations, especially about art. It's a sketch of Dr. Patel—a flattering caricature. His exaggeratedly large head has an unmistakeable resemblance, whereas his diminutive body appears to be that of a body builder. He's flexing both arms and looks proud. The pencil lines and shading are impressive.

Dr. Patel turns, and then turns back to me, grinning. His smile seemed mischievous when I met him in the ER, but today I see delight. I understand now that mania distorted my view of many people at that time. Dr. Patel has helped me so much—he met me at my worst and has kindly put up with me ever since. It is nice to see his smile. It reassures me that he's not out to get me, he's only ever wanted to help me. As usual, the anticipation of these appointments is more nerve-wracking than the actual meeting itself. Still, I can't let my guard down. I offer a measured smile in return.

"Yes," he says. "Tell me, what do you think the artist's diagnosis is?"

I contemplate his question for a moment that stretches out too long. Will he make a note that I'm not capable of answering simple questions? My palms start to sweat.

"I don't know. Crazy?"

His face remains fixed with a joyful grin. I don't think he likes that word, possibly he's been taught not to use that stigmatized, overused, derogatory word, but he doesn't flinch.

"Mania."

The word hangs in the air between us like a noose. I don't know anyone else with bipolar disorder and seeing art produced by someone like me, someone in the throes of manic creativity, hits me in my throat. I have no desire to connect to other manic people because I don't want to be a part of this club. Dr. Patel breaks the silence by describing the meaning behind each part of the drawing, because of course each pencil stroke has meaning. Manic people do everything with intention, especially when it comes to art. I am fascinated, despite my mild repulsion.

"It is a terrible, terrible disease," he says.

Disease? Is this a disease? I thought it was an illness. Disease sounds so much worse. And, terrible? How can something be terrible when it produces such inspired art? I guess he's seen more terrible things than I can imagine, but does that justify such a broad label? Last May was terrible for me and Eric, and our family, but since then it hasn't been so bad. I wouldn't say it's as terrible as cancer. Or a miscarriage. Or possibly even severe asthma. Or so many other things that people have to endure. I open my mouth to respond, to tell Dr. Patel that it's not as terrible as he thinks, but then I remember that I'm not supposed to argue. I'm not supposed to question him or any of the experts. That could be interpreted as a lack of trust. Paranoia. I close my mouth.

"So, Charise, how are you feeling?"

He picks up his pen and we move on to the purpose of the visit. I put the sketch and our difference of opinions out of my mind. I answer his questions honestly, which is easy to do because they are very straightforward. How much I've been sleeping (eight hours per night), how my moods have been (stable with mild vacation excitement and general winter fatigue), how is Eric (good), the usual. Dr. Patel says he wishes Eric were here today. Not because he thinks I need support or might be lying, he just likes talking to Eric. I find this annoying, but I'm not allowed to be irritable. Eric has been great, but what about me? I'm the one doing the work, changing my life, staying on track. I wish he would throw me a bone once in a while.

"Have you had any new side effects to the medication?"

I stare blankly before shaking my head. How would I know if I've experienced side effects? When I look online, it seems like anything can be a side effect: mild thirst, frequent urination, hand tremors, drowsiness, weight gain, lightheadedness, nausea, diarrhea, lack of awareness, clumsiness, ringing in the ears, vomiting, confusion, difficulty walking, blue colour in extremities, poor memory, seizures, muscle weakness, and depression. Last fall I asked him if lithium changes my tastebuds because everything tasted dull. He shrugged it off like it was impossible, which makes me reluctant to ask about other things. I think my medication is responsible for many things, like my acne flare-ups, but I can't be certain. Nothing feels severe enough to ask or complain about and besides, I have to stay on the meds. At least for now.

"Do you think I'm still on track to start weaning off in the spring?" I say.

He nods.

"Yes, everything looks all right. We'll see at the one year mark."

The one year mark is three months away. I can do three more months.

"How are you spending your days, Charise?"

I work to control my facial expression. My daughter is in half-day kindergarten, which means that between school drop-offs and pick-ups I get less than two hours to myself every day. Two hours to squeeze in a workout and a small amount of writing. What is it about taking care of children, a house, a dog, and myself that this man does not understand? Does he think I'm a lady who lunches in between yoga and mani-pedis?

"I'm with Suzie most of the time. And I have a lot of family obligations." I can see that my answer does not please him. Being a housewife is never enough. "I've been volunteering at my children's school."

He starts to nod. This answer he likes.

"I'm thinking of looking for work again," I say. Helping with school lunches and coaxing reluctant students to read does not feel as rewarding as job productivity and a paycheque.

A wrinkle passes over Dr. Patel's forehead. I shouldn't have mentioned it.

"You tried that and it didn't work." He peers up while writing notes about me. His statement is more matter-of-fact than unkind, but I'm taken aback. Just because I tried once, a week after being released from a psych ward, I should never try again?

"Maybe more volunteering," I say with a weak voice. He nods again. He seems pleased that I want to do something, just not something that takes up too much time. Adds too much stress.

"Do you know any mental health organizations other than OBAD where I could volunteer?"

OBAD is the Organization for Bipolar Affective Disorder. I browsed their website for volunteer opportunities but currently there are none. I have never attended their support group meetings or workshops, although I should. I loved group therapy and peer support after my miscarriage, so many years ago. The hardest part was admitting I needed help, but those meetings saved me. I'm not sure why I'm reluctant to join OBAD—the connection with similarly struggling people could be beneficial. Maybe it's because this doesn't feel nearly as hard as my miscarriage.

"No," Dr. Patel says. He offers nothing more. Doesn't he like the idea of me doing meaningful volunteer work? Maybe he thinks I'm not capable or qualified to help people with mental health problems, just like I'm not capable of working.

He finishes writing another sentence about me and puts his pen down. He looks up, making eye contact, and the quiet between us grows heavy as we wait for each other to speak.

"You could volunteer to be a greeter downstairs," he finally says.

"A greeter?" I ask. "The person who says hello at the door?"

He nods and elaborates on how fulfilling it is, as though he himself has tried it and found pleasure in the position. He talks about how critical it is for me to find meaning in my life. I was a robotics engineer for fifteen years. How will standing around talking to passersby provide meaning? From what I've seen, this role is performed by older people, those who have worked their whole lives and need a retirement hobby. Is this all he thinks I'm capable of, being put out to pasture? I may as well get a job at Tim Horton's, at least then I'd make minimum wage.

I hesitate, wanting to share my broader aspirations—writing, art, a master's degree—but not sure if revealing such passion will get me in trouble. I decide to speak up. I can't leave this appointment on such a low note.

"I've been writing," I say. Dr. Patel's eyebrows shoot up in an expression of surprise. His mouth remains flat.

"Really?" He picks up his pen. "What are you writing?"

I elaborate about my book, which started out as therapeutic journaling and quickly grew into something more. I reveal small details slowly, and he listens patiently, prompting me to continue each time I pause, as though he is reeling in a line to coax a fish from the water. I have kept this passion of mine secret because I don't know if he will see my creativity as psychotic—another symptom, another delusion. He scribbles while I talk. Good or bad notations, I'll never know. When I finish, he nods his head but says nothing about all that I've just revealed. No wonder he likes my husband so much. They are so similar, and both like to hold their cards close to their chests.

"Well, Charise, your numbers look good. Your lithium levels are perfect. Your thyroid is functioning well. Everything looks good," he says. Our conversation has reached its natural conclusion. "Whatever you're doing, keep doing it."

This makes me feel proud. Finally, some acknowledgment for my hard work! That's the bone I wanted him to throw me.

"Tell Eric I said hello. And bring him next time."

He laughs and I smile. This time his request feels prickly, because he is no longer asking for a visit from Eric simply to socialize. He wants to hear Eric's opinion of me and my mental health before assessing if we can reduce my lithium. Dr. Patel's seemingly casual comment reminds me that no matter how I present myself, how calm and sane I appear to be, he will always value Eric's version of events more than my own. Eric's word will be taken as the truth when our accounts differ, no matter what I say. But I'm willing to put on a show for the few remaining moments until I can walk out of this room, out of this hospital, and back into the cold Calgary sunshine. Anything to get back to lunch with my daughter, our house, and my apparently unfulfilling family life. Anything to get away from this place.

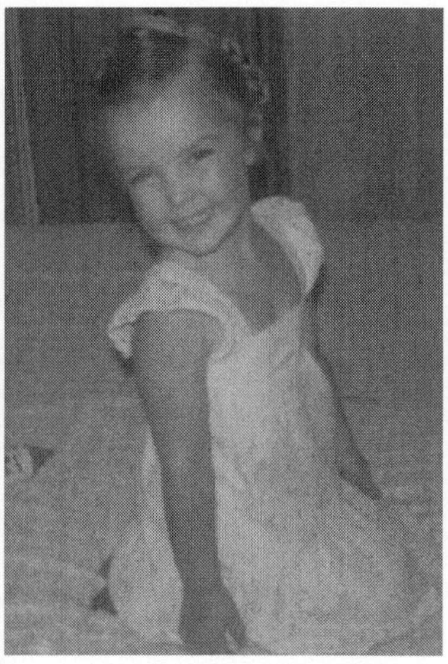

Three years old, 1980.

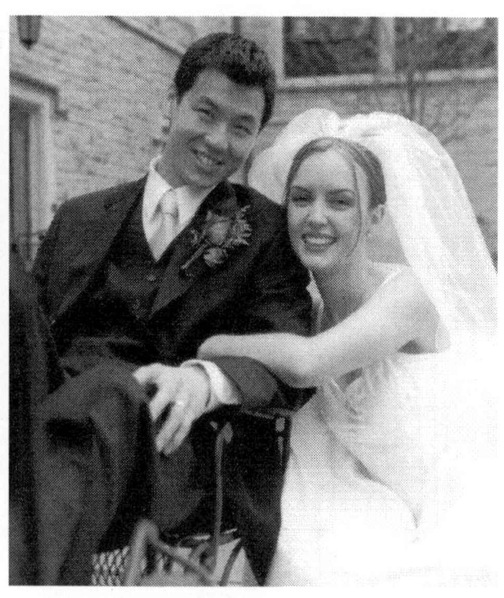

Our wedding, April 2002.

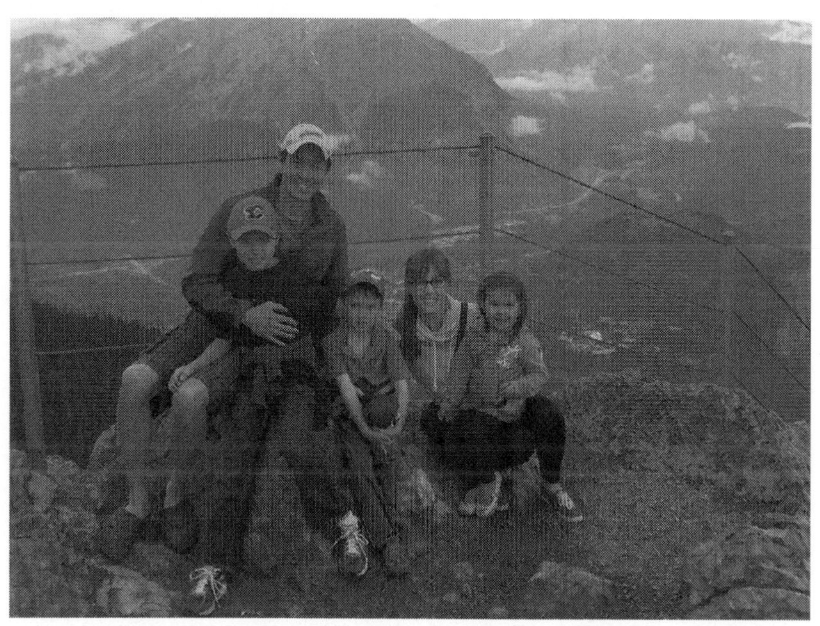

This picture was taken a few weeks after we moved to Calgary in 2015. We loved to explore and embraced our new home.

Pre-hospitalization
Early May 2017

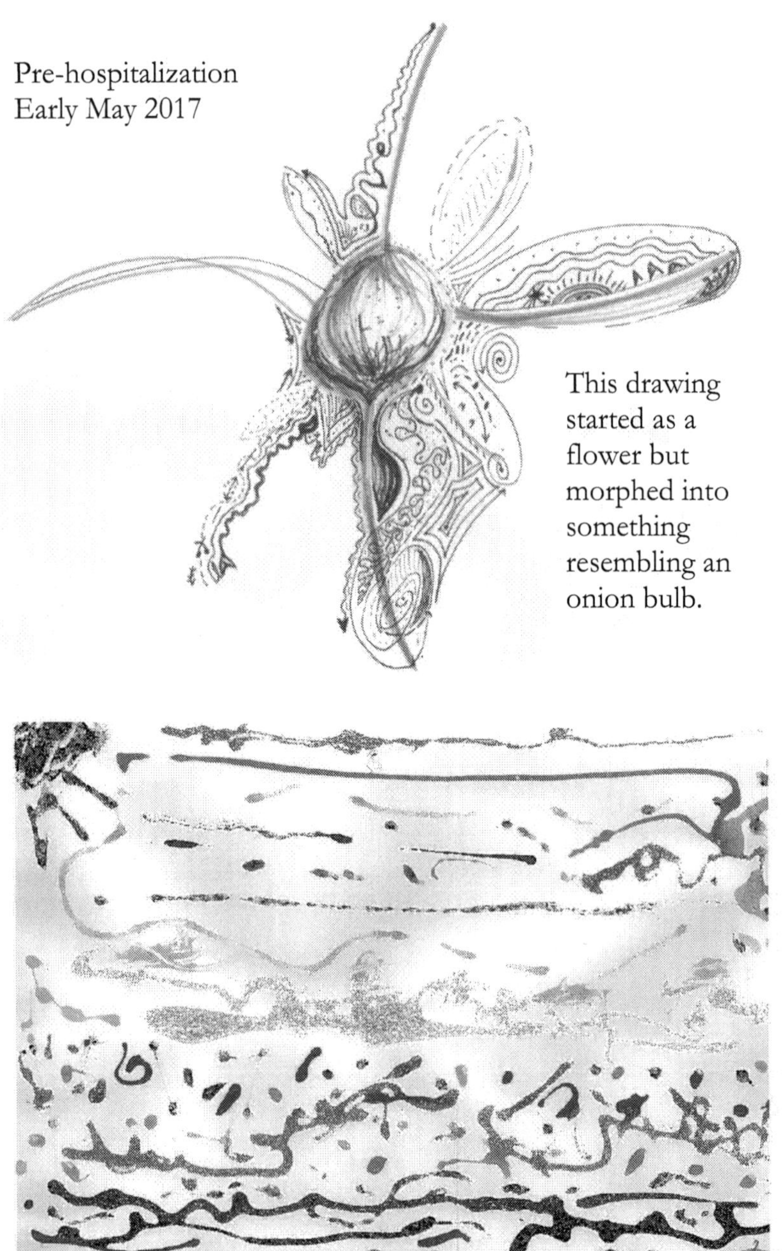

This drawing started as a flower but morphed into something resembling an onion bulb.

My art became more abstract as I became more manic. Here, I used my daughter's glitter pens to quickly sketch the view of the snow-capped mountains. It was a sunny day.

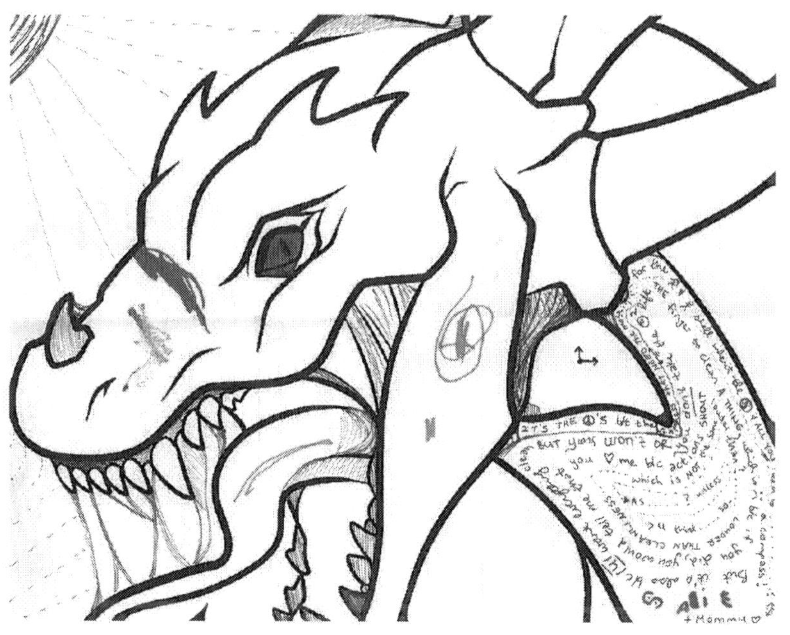


Psych ward art: dragons and my northern lights river.

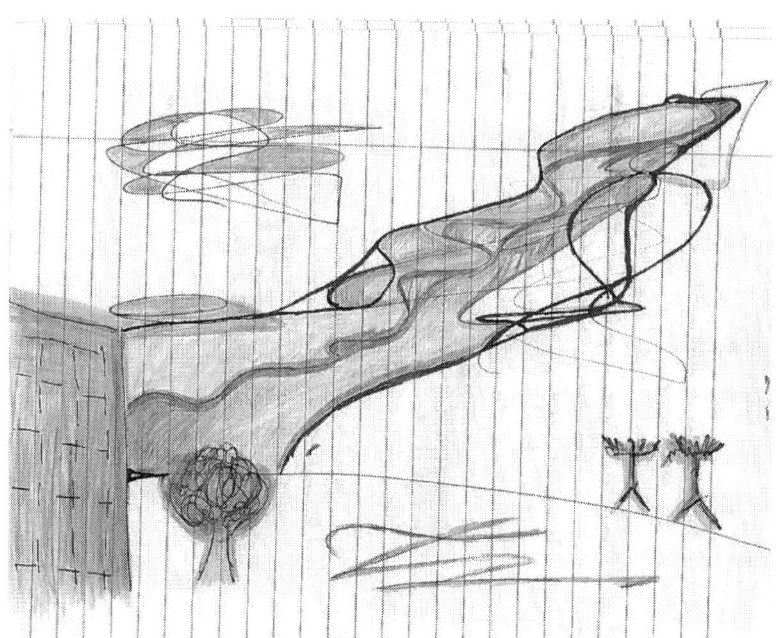

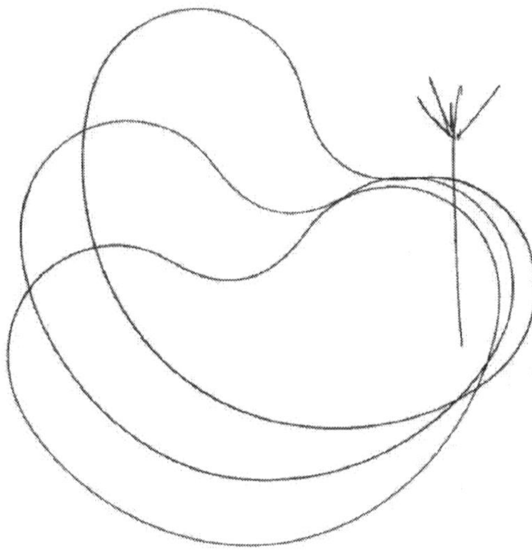

After being released from the hospital, I drew this simple Picasso Peace Dove with a stencil for my children. It was wonderful to feel artistic again.

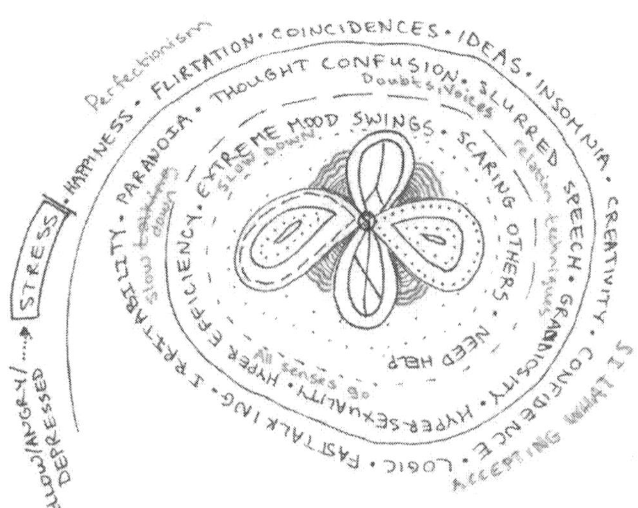


This was me trying to break down the initial symptoms of my manic episode with the later ones, and determine where they crossed the line.

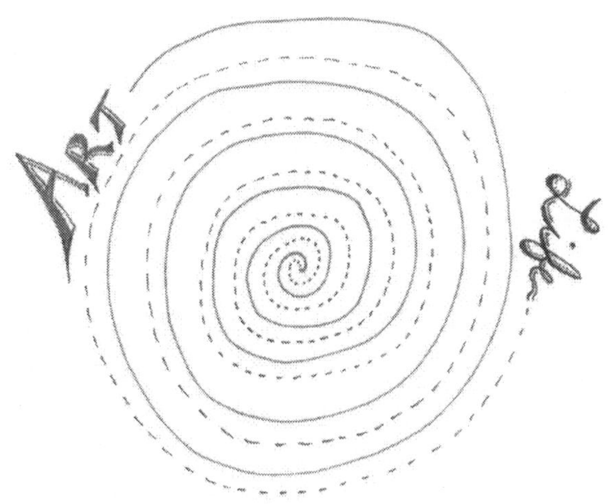


By late 2017, I wanted so much to create beautiful art, but I was uninspired and had no confidence in my abilities.

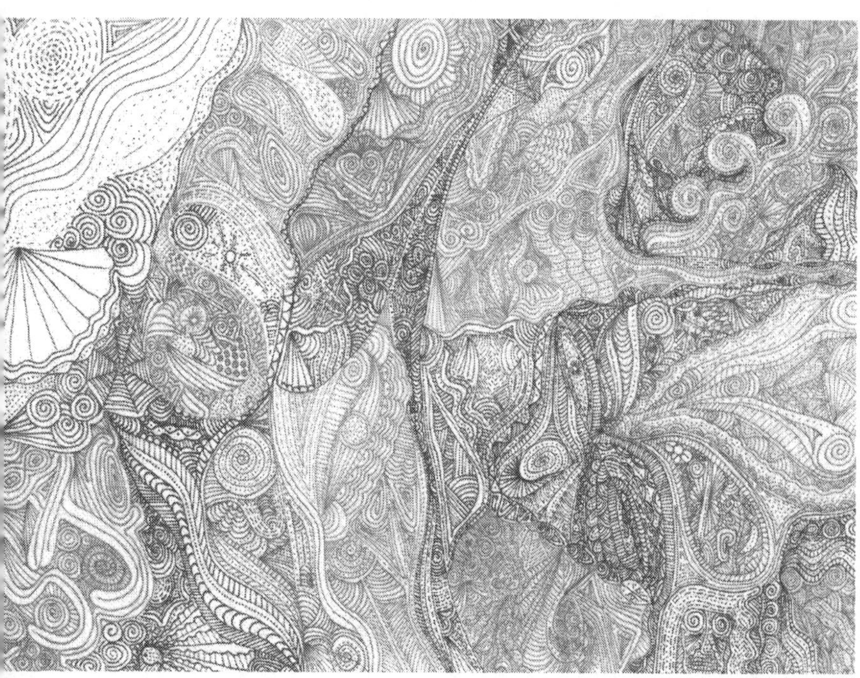

My children informed me that this art technique is called zentangling. I didn't know it was a thing, I just wanted to draw. This felt therapeutic.

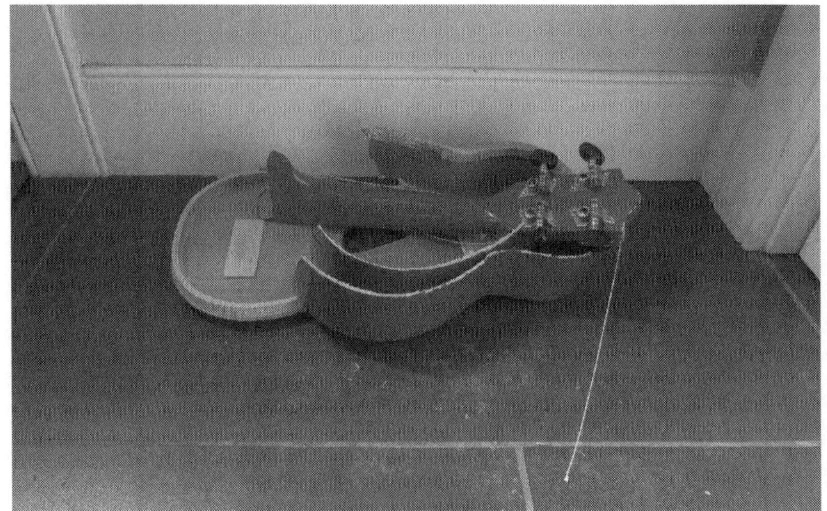

Eric broke our ukulele in frustration because I reduced my medication in 2018. I took a picture to prove that I'm not the only person who gets angry, just the only one who gets hospitalized because of it. I also thought the broken ukulele looked artistic.

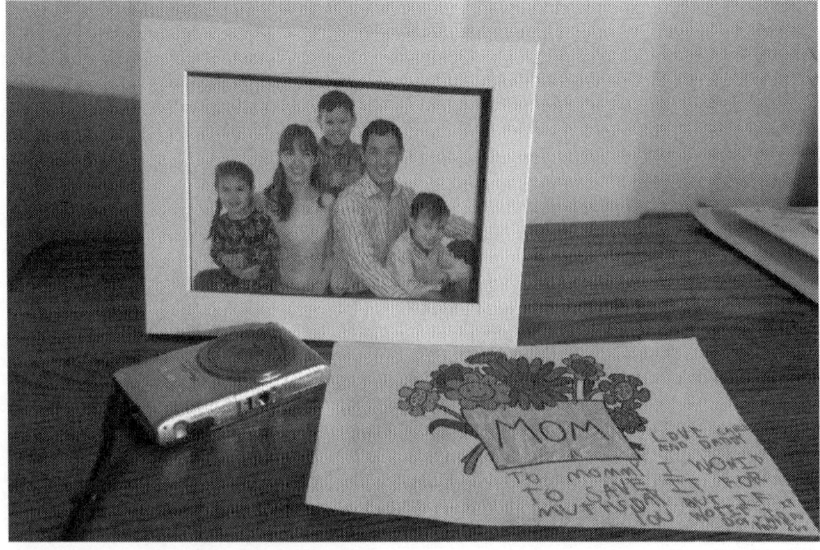


Suzie gave me this Mother's Day card early, in case I had to go to the hospital because of my manic symptoms. It was wise: I was raging in the ER on Mother's Day. This is the family photograph that got broken when I was assaulted by the security guard.

2018 psych ward art. Spirals and colours appeal to me during mania. This picture started as a way for me to express my rage and helped me work through many difficult emotions.

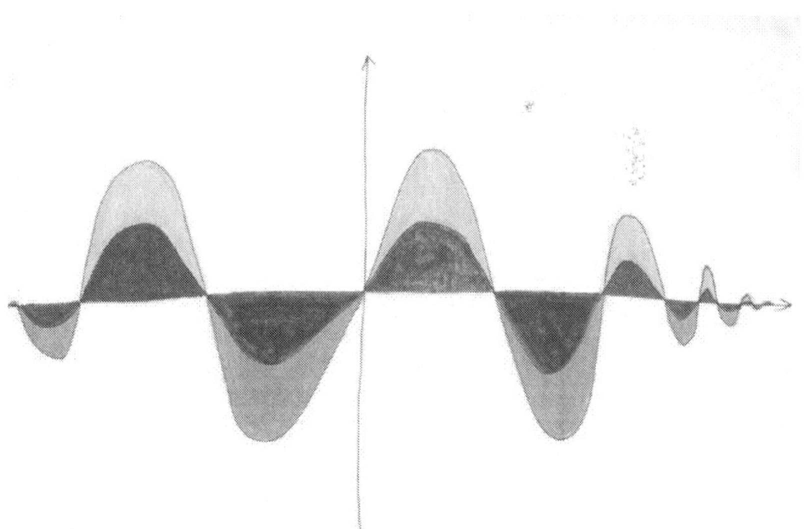

I likened my mania and depression to a sine curve, with the top half of the graph being mania and the bottom half, depression.

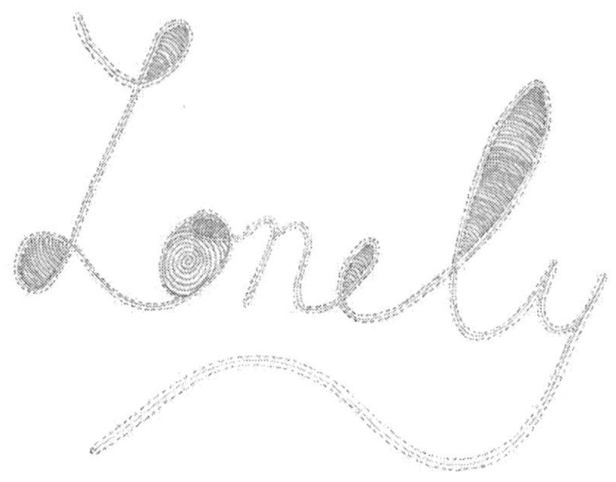


More doodle-sketching to express how I felt.

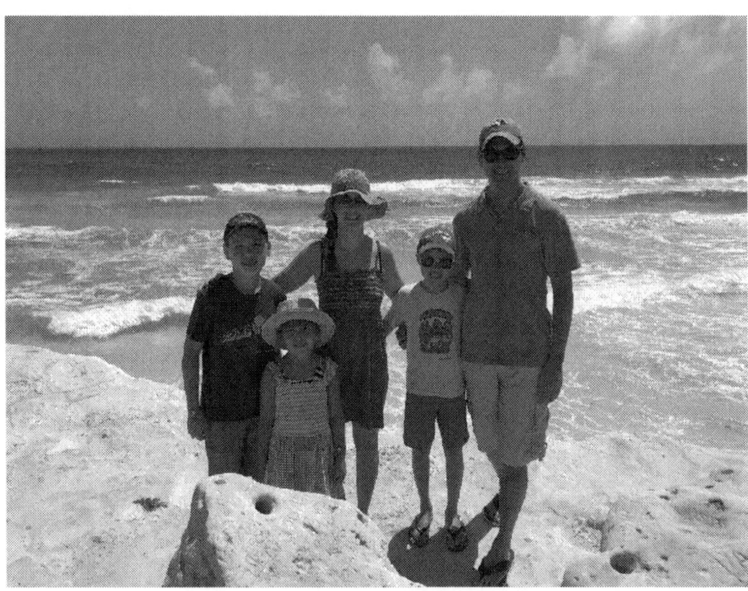

Mexico, March, 2019. Eric and I were both concerned about another spring manic episode and hospitalization, but it was a fantastic vacation.

# 24. Cruising

This multi-family cruise was a great idea, especially since April in Alberta can still be brutally cold. Mom and Dad should arrive any minute—they must be so excited. We landed in Florida yesterday, but they are driving from Toronto, which takes longer than flying from Calgary. My sister and her family arrive tomorrow. We'll all board the ship together.

"Okay, guys, Nona just texted to say they're close," I say. Suzie rests on my hip with my arms wrapped around her. Her brothers stand too close to the curb outside the hotel, watching for my parents' car.

"I see them!" Jack says. Alex starts to wave. Suzie is too tired to respond. The two hour time difference has thrown her off. She snuggles into my neck and I feel her eyelashes brush my skin. I take the opportunity to sniff her forehead and hair, and squeeze her close. I won't be able to do this for much longer. I can barely carry her now that she's five.

"Great," I say, but I'm skeptical. Both boys have claimed sightings a number of times already. But then I see the car that Jack and Alex are pointing to, my mom's profile in the passenger seat, and my dad's smile as he drives through the parking lot towards us.

"Alex, Jack, back up!" I'm excited but also concerned about one of the boys eagerly darting out towards the car.

They obediently move back while waving and jumping up and down. Suzie lifts her head, curiosity replacing exhaustion. Dad pulls up beside us and rolls down his window.

"Hi, guys," he says calmly despite his huge grin.

"Hi, Pops!" Jack and Alex run to pat his arm, hold his hand, and be as close as they can get with his car door between them.

"Popsie!" Suzie says. She is now fully awake and squirming to get down. I slide her to the ground but keep a tight hold on her hand.

"Great to see you," I say with a wide smile. "How was the drive?"

"Oh, fine, thanks."

Mom leans forward to talk and wave, but then decides she can't wait. She releases her seatbelt, opens her door, steps out of the car, and runs around the front to join us on the sidewalk. She squeezes us all into a tight hug, and everybody squeezes her back.

"It's so good to see you guys!"

She has tears in her eyes and her smile radiates pure joy. The kids huddle around her legs, clamouring for attention. We all talk at the same time.

"You should have seen the look on your face when you saw us, Nona!"

"I lost a tooth on the plane!"

"Are you excited for the boat?"

All I can think is *thank God.* Thank God for my parents.

"Do you want to go across the hall to show Nona and Pops and your cousins?" I say to Jack and Suzie. They are delighted with their ship-supplied eye patches and bandanas, the only pirate gear we have because I did not pack anything for tonight's themed dinner. My sister told me to bring costumes months ago. I forgot. Looking at my woefully underdressed children, I realize that I should have paid attention. Maybe a better mom would have brought swords and earrings and even a parrot. Maybe my children deserve that better mom, the one who cares a little more about this bullshit. When I have these thoughts, I wonder if I'm falling into the depression side of bipolar or if it's just standard mom guilt. I look again at their smiles. They are delighted to wear free "costumes," and I am reminded that this is what it's all about. Raising happy, healthy, honest, good people who aren't spoiled.

They eagerly leave our room to cross the hall to visit my parents. I hear them knock loudly, but our door slams shut before the opposite door is opened. I listen until I hear my mom's voice welcoming them inside.

I turn to look at Eric. He has been lying on our bed in this tiny cabin for an hour. To be fair, there isn't anywhere else for him to relax. Jack and Suzie share the bunkbed that lines the hallway, which takes away the pull-out couch seating area. There is a small vanity table housing a TV and our clutter. It has a chair, which is unusable while the couch is in bed form. So, Eric is on our bed. Lately he has been on his phone or watching TV, but now when I look, he is asleep. Typical. We're supposed to be in the dining room in half an hour. I inhale and exhale deeply, and shake my head. I don't know what is going on with him, but it is annoying. Maybe it's because we're vacationing with my family. Or I'm not paying him enough attention. Or the trip is expensive, he had to leave his tequila in the car, the cabin was disappointing, and there's no volleyball court. Maybe his attitude has nothing to do with me, the trip, or anything at all. Maybe he's just moody. Lucky for him that he won't be committed.

I'm not going to let him wreck my fun. I haven't seen my parents in a year and I want to enjoy every minute. I feel great. I haven't felt any side effects from cutting back my stupid lithium before we left. I debated self-weaning for weeks, but Dr. Patel said I could only do it under his supervision at the one year mark. There are many reasons why I want off it (I think it's a placebo, I don't know the long-term consequences, I managed without it for forty years, it makes my acne worse, it takes away my creativity, I can't concentrate, and overall life is way less fun), but the main reason is that I don't like medication. I don't want to be dependent on drugs. I held out as long as I could—until just three weeks shy of one year, and then I cut back to two-thirds of my regular dosage. 600mg instead of 900mg. I haven't told anybody. I'll tell them after my experiment works.

The only problem is that my sleep hasn't been great, but I attribute that to being in stuffy hotel rooms and then a tomblike cruise ship cabin, plus the time change, so I'm not worried. I slept poorly in Mexico a few months ago and didn't go manic, so I'm sure it's just a vacation thing. I am grouchy and irritable, yes, but that's normal for anyone a little sleep deprived. I am definitely not hypersexual since Eric's being such a jerk, and I haven't had any manic euphoria or energy. My acne is clearing up, and I feel lighter without the drugs coursing through my body. I can't wait to cut back even more, and I really can't wait to cut it out entirely. I knew it was a good idea. I knew I didn't need to wait three more weeks for Dr. Patel's permission and supervision. I am not a child.

"So what if she doesn't like dogs?"

It's the last night of our vacation. We're stuck at another airless hotel until we fly out tomorrow, and I am once again unable to sleep. After fitfully wrestling with my thoughts for hours, Eric woke up and asked if I was okay. Somehow his concern led us here, to yet another random argument.

"What makes you think you're such a perfect parent?" I say.

"I never said I was a perfect parent. I think if I see a problem and know how to help then it's my duty to help."

"What duty? Your sister never asked for help. Nobody likes unsolicited advice, especially about parenting."

Eric pulls his hand away from its resting spot on my stomach. I'm surprised that it's stayed there this long. He puts both hands under his pillow, under his head. I feel his watchful glare, but I stare at the ceiling, eyes locked on nothing in an effort to avoid looking at him. Finally, the silence between us is too great. I turn towards him.

"What?" I say.

"Why are you so mad at me?"

It sounds like an innocent question. He's good at asking questions that sound innocent. I can never tell if it's because he sincerely wants to know the answer, or because he's learned that pretending to care will make me more sympathetic. It will shut me up faster.

"I'm mad because this whole vacation you've been so moody. So particular. Everything had to be your way and when it wasn't you just couldn't accommodate anyone else," I say.

"I couldn't accommodate anyone else? This whole trip has been about your family! All I've done is accommodate everyone else!"

"That's a cop-out."

Our eyes have been locked together but now he breaks contact and flips onto his back. I can see him roll his eyes despite the darkness.

"When we were in that movie theatre on the ship the kids were so excited. You didn't want to stay, so you just left," I say, to prove my point.

"I didn't want to watch the movie. It was stupid."

"You think I did? We were there for the kids. They wanted you there but because it wasn't convenient for you, you took off."

"So that's why I ruined the vacation, because I didn't want to watch a movie?"

"I never said you ruined the vacation."

"You said I was moody and wouldn't accommodate anyone."

"You were," I say. I glance at the alarm clock on the night stand. We have to leave in four hours, drive to the airport, and fly back home, and I'm nowhere near sleep.

"This morning at breakfast," I say. "You stood up to leave before anyone else was finished. When you put your backpack on the strap whipped around and hit me in the eye. It stung so badly, and you didn't even notice. My dad was trying to help me but we were rushing to keep up with you, so I couldn't even take a minute to recuperate."

"I didn't know that." He turns to look at me. "Are you okay? I didn't know it hit you."

"Of course you didn't. Every time you snap your fingers and we have to follow, and you never look back. When we boarded the ship

Jack got in trouble by the crew because he was trying to keep up with you and you were too far ahead."

"I never knew that happened."

"That's my point! You don't turn around. You assume we're fine and I've got the rear. You leave a movie or a meal with no awareness."

"I didn't know that happened. I'm sorry the strap hit you. I didn't mean for it to hit you. There was a window of time for us to leave the ship before it got chaotic."

He's either not listening or not hearing. Since when did we stop seeing things eye-to-eye? Why does this have to be so difficult?

"Mommy, I need the bathroom," Suzie says. We are in an airport lounge, waiting to board our flight home.

"Okay, sweetie," I say. I lift my purse and do a quick check to make sure it contains my wallet and phone. "Let's go."

We stand. I survey the scene. We were amongst the earlier travellers to arrive but now most of the chairs are full. Eric and the boys sit in nearby seats, each one of them craning their necks down to play on a device.

"Suzie and I are going to the bathroom," I say, to no one in particular. Eric glances up momentarily to nod an acknowledgement or perhaps his permission, I don't know. Whatever. I am still furious about our unresolved argument. So furious that I decide to text my sister. I want evidence to prove my point. And for validation. I reach into my purse with one hand while holding Suzie's hand tightly with the other, and as we weave through the chairs and travellers, and dodge airport travel carts on our way to the bathroom, I compose a text asking my sister if she thought Eric behaved like a child throwing a tantrum during the trip.

Suzie and I go into adjacent stalls and she automatically starts to sing. I trained her to do this so we wouldn't have to share a stall and I wouldn't have to worry about somebody snatching her. As long as I can hear her voice, I know she's safe. I'm almost in a good mood because of her song when I hear my phone ping. I quickly reach for it and read my sister's response.

"Not really."

She's written more, but those are the only two words that resonate. My body instantly clenches. She must not have seen it. But how could she not have, when there were so many times he stormed off? Why aren't either of them acknowledging it? Have they had some kind of conversation about me, like they did last year? Are Mom and Dad in on it too? Is everybody talking about me again?

Suzie has stopped singing, so I call her name as I quickly finish up and open the door, my pulse starting to race. She stands three feet away, diligently washing her hands, proud of herself for beating me to the sink. She turns to smile when she sees my reflection in the mirror. Suzie is radiant, as usual. I join her and focus on this moment, not whatever is going on with my husband and my family behind my back.

"I beat you!" Suzie says with a grin.

"You sure did," I say. We play with our soap bubbles and I enjoy other women's adoring gazes and compliments. As Suzie rubs her hands together and splashes the water, I run my fingers through my long hair to nimbly weave the strands into a casual over-the-shoulder braid that somehow manages to look exquisite despite its simplicity. I realized last May, just before my manic episode, that the countless times I'd braided Suzie's hair had trained my fingers to do my own. Seemingly overnight I could reach the back and sides of my head to create French braids and fish tails without a mirror or a moment's pause. I stopped braiding my hair after being released from the hospital because the medication made me less coordinated. The few times I tried were frustrating and the result was disappointing. And then I forgot about this hairstyle that pleases Eric, and most of the men, so much. I'm not sure what happened but something on the cruise reminded me of the braids. I guess I like to look pretty when I'm exhausted just as much as I like to look sexy when I'm manic. This last thought makes me pause to reconsider this elaborate hairstyle I've just created with ease, and for a moment I wonder if I should be concerned. But then I notice how happy Suzie looks and I push the thought from my mind.

When we finish playing and preening, Suzie uses the paper towel she dried her hands with to open the door, just like I taught her, and holds it open for me. I wave an elderly woman through ahead of us.

"What a sweetheart! Thank you dear," she says to Suzie, who doesn't know how to respond and starts to blush. I take her hand and we follow behind the woman. On the way back to our gate, we pass a David's Tea. I slow down to take a closer look at the boxes on display.

"I like the colours," Suzie says. We stop and point out which boxes we find the most appealing. There are all kinds at all price points, but the one that catches both of our eyes is the Mother's Day box, right at the very top. It's elegant and calming, filled with a variety of tea bags with refreshing, relaxing names. It is everything a mother would want for Mother's Day, if she likes tea. I like tea. And I'm a mother. I learnt years ago to buy a present for myself for Mother's Day, or my birthday, or Valentine's Day, to recognize and honour myself. And also, it would be a nice treat to feel better about all this crap going on with Eric. Should I buy it? I definitely want it and Mother's Day is coming up, but it's twenty-four dollars. For tea. And also, if I buy it, will it be interpreted as manic shopping? Could it be manic shopping? No, it's just tea. I think.

"I kind of want to buy it," I say even as I implore my stubborn feet to start walking again. They feel rooted into the tiles of this airport hallway.

"You should, Mommy," Suzie says.

"It's a lot of money though," I say.

"Oh," she says, which doesn't help me. She starts to grow restless waiting for me to make a decision.

"Mommy, look at all that makeup!"

I look where she's pointing, across the aisle at a MAC cosmetics shop, and my heart skips a beat. Will I be tempted to splurge on makeup now? Will I want to get dressed up again and start to be hypersexual? Could I be going manic? We have to get out of here.

I step away from temptation and guide my daughter back toward our waiting area. Along the way, I notice many looks of admiration from the men we pass, just like this time last year. I know it is not my imagination. It is as real now as it was then. I force a smile, as though I'm having so much fun with Suzie that I would rather be here than anywhere else, which is true. We have a lot of fun together. I have a lot of fun with each of my kids. But my smile doesn't say that. It is a mask. My attempt to push away the fear that's starting to creep into my exhausted brain. My smile is returned by every single person that we pass, men and women alike. How often does that happen in an airport? Could this be a delusion? Surely not. Suzie smiles too, so maybe that's all it is. Maybe they're not attracted to me, they are merely admiring a happy and sweet mother and daughter in these dreary, tiring surroundings. Yes, that's it, we're a sight for sore eyes. And I resisted the tea, so that's good. And the braid is just a braid, a way to keep my hair out of the way, nothing more. I've got this under control.

We sit down beside the boys, who don't lift their eyes from their screens, and I hand Suzie her iPad. I'm too tired to interact further. I pull out my phone for a distraction. I find the Crossword app and press to open it, but instead of going into puzzles like it normally does, a screen appears that says, "Welcome Mother of Dragons." My breath catches in my throat. Seems like the universe is trying to send me a message, just like last May. Fuck.

# 25. The Art / Life Blur

I hear a key in the lock and the handle turns. Eric opens the back door and steps into the mudroom adjacent to the kitchen. I look up from my seat at the table. I'm excited to see him, I have so much to tell him, but I'm too busy to stop. I'll have to take a break.

"Hi, handsome!" I stand and walk over to greet him. He's letting cold air into our warm, cozy house. He wrestles with his hockey bag and eventually pulls it inside. He rests his stick against the wall beside the boot tray.

"Hi, Reese." He kisses my cheek. "You're so hot."

I smile. I'm wearing fleece pyjamas, and have had the fire burning for hours, but that's not why I'm hot. It's because of my work. Physical work makes me hot. Now I realize that mental work has the same result.

"I've done so much," I say. He hands me his water bottle and I place it on the counter. "I haven't been inspired like this since last spring! I can't get my ideas down fast enough!"

"That's great," he says without enthusiasm. It's more than great. It's amazing! One of the worst things about those stupid drugs was how they blocked my ideas. I haven't been creative at all. I wonder how inspired I'll be when I'm totally weaned. I can't wait!

"How was your game?" I say.

He goes into detail and I try to pay attention but my mind drifts. It's too far away to bring it back.

"Were you writing?"

I nod.

"A new series. I've figured so much out." I look to my notebook on the kitchen table. "It's all coming together. I just have a bit more to do and then I'll show you."

I walk back to the table and pick up my pencil. I've almost got everything resolved. Eric takes his hockey gear away and then I hear the shower. I'm so immersed in my work that I barely notice when he returns with his laptop.

"Okay if I sit here?" he asks. My papers are spread all over the table. I nod and make space. I'm almost ready to pack it up anyway, I just need to finish the sleep-rest yin yang. He sets up his laptop, spreads out his legal pad and supplies, and starts to type. And then he stops.

"Can we talk about Toronto?"

"What about it?" I say, distracted.

"Do you still think it's a good idea?"

A few days ago, Eric's boss asked him to move back to Toronto—to pack our family up and move back, less than three years after he asked him to pack our family up and move here. I think we already decided to say yes.

"Sure," I say. "Don't you?"

He nods. He stares at me with intensity.

"I want to be sure you're okay with it," he says.

I cock my head and glance up at the ceiling.

"Absolutely. We'll be back with family and friends, it's helpful for your career, and maybe I get my job back. Sounds good."

He pauses. It's clear that there's something more he wants to say but he is the strong, silent type. I can't coax anything from him. I wait for a moment but I'm not in the mood to be patient. I've got work to do.

"Anything else?" I say.

"No," he says. "Just checking." He pauses between each word as though to give me an opportunity to interrupt. To take back my reassurances that moving to Toronto will be fine. But everything with us is always fine, so why would I take it back?

"Okay." I pick up my pencil and return to my words. But they're not coming anymore. I've lost the inspiration. I doodle, hoping that I'll remember what I was about to write, with no success.

"Are you working?" I say. Eric nods absentmindedly. It's uncharacteristic of him to work this late on a typical night, and this week was supposed to be lighter. Because of me.

"Didn't you say you were working less, just in case?" I'm still not sleeping well since our vacation threw me off. And men are noticing me. I think I'm okay, but just in case, I've implemented rules based on what excited me too much last spring: I'm only putting on subtle makeup, doing simple hairstyles, no jewelry aside from my wedding ring. I'm not shopping except for groceries, I write and speak slowly with proper enunciation, I don't talk too much, no using symbol shortcuts instead of a written word, no taking photos of inanimate objects that look artistic, no more than one photograph per day, no more than one social media post per day, no friendly chit-chat with strangers, no flirting, no lingerie, and do not under any circumstances be alone with a man other than my psychiatrist or husband. Rules are the only way I know to suppress my instincts. This is my best Fake-It-Until-You-Make-It approach for hypomania, the milder form of mania that can lead to a full-blown manic episode.

"Yes. But now I have to work."

His tone is cold, or he's distracted. I'm confused. According to him he wasn't planning to work much until we're out of the woods. Yet now he has to work? Confused doesn't describe what I feel. Suspicious, doubtful, paranoid—that's more like it.

I decide I'm done for today. I was supposed to start winding down half an hour ago and will never fall asleep if I don't start relaxing now.

"Do you want to watch something?" I stand and collect my sketches and notes. After sorting them into an organized stack, I carefully bang the edges on the table to align them in a perfect rectangle. I then place them on my closed laptop and move the pile to the dining room, which now doubles as my office. I'm not sure what motivated me to write in the kitchen tonight. I never do. But then, I rarely write at night anymore either. It stimulates my insomnia.

I pick up the remote and drop onto the couch. I don't know if Eric replied, but he's still at the table, so I don't think he's joining me. I'm still perplexed about his sudden urgent work. It's highly atypical.

Flipping through Netflix, I spot a movie that I've noticed before. *Anon.* I'm intrigued. I press play and am overwhelmed by the realistic imagery that appears on the screen. It feels intense and confusing. I can't follow the storyline even though I think it's about me. The actors stare into me when they speak, and before long I start answering their questions. I swivel to look at Eric. He is on high alert, as we approach the one-year mark of my Mother's Day mania, so if I'm talking to movie characters who are talking to me, he'll notice. He hasn't yet, so he must still be focused on his work. I'm still safe from him overreacting. I'm not too far gone yet that I can't come back on my own. At least, I don't think so. I just feel really good. But if Eric starts to pay too much attention then everything I do will be under a microscope and sooner or later I'll be in the hospital again. I have to rein it in. I have to be calm.

The movie demands my attention. I'm so overwhelmed that I can't remain seated. I stand and begin to pace, speaking loudly. I don't know the characters' names—those particulars escaped me early on—so I use the actors' names. I don't think they'll mind. I only know Clive and Colm, so the rest of them become 'buddy,' 'the girl,' or something equally vague. I can't remember what happened at the beginning, I only know that I'm very frustrated. Pacing, I turn and see that Eric has stopped working. He's closed his laptop and is staring straight at me. Hard. He looks concerned, sad, and apprehensive.

"Reese, I think we should turn off the TV," he says slowly.

I shrug. I couldn't care less. Remarkable considering how invested I felt a moment ago. I continue to pace in circles, but I slow down. Eric picks up the remote and shuts everything off. He then pulls me next to him and we both collapse onto the couch, me wrapped tightly in his arms. I'm not sure why he's suddenly so affectionate, but I like it.

"Did you take your lithium?" he asks.

I pause. I have a system to remember if I've taken my meds but right now I forget what it is.

"Yes," I say. I'm not sure I did but I'd rather keep up appearances. I once asked Dr. Patel what to do if I forgot to take them before bed, and he said to take them the next night. So, even if I didn't take them tonight surely one night won't make much of a difference. Besides, I'll be cutting them out completely soon enough. A few more weeks at 600mg and I can drop to 300mg.

"Okay, good. We should get to bed."

Easy for him to say. For him, getting to bed means falling asleep.

"Okay."

He kisses my forehead, a soft, tender kiss, and then pulls me to a standing position. I hope my plan works. I hope I sleep tonight. I hope I don't have to go the hospital. I hope everything will be okay.

## 26. Repercussions

The dread in my core grows with each passing second. I take a deep breath and remind myself that this is for the best. That I should do the next right thing, as Clint Malarchuk would say.A memory appears from last spring: I'm crying and raging in the psych ward. It is effective. It gets my feet to move, one in front of the other, down the stairs. Anything to prevent that nightmare. Eric told me last year that he kept saying, "She's not wrong," to others when discussing something I'd said or emailed while manic. It made me feel so supported and loved. I hold onto that memory hopefully as I creep down the stairs towards my unassuming husband whom, with any luck, I will find fast asleep on the couch.

The television's blue light shines down the hall. I stealthily tiptoe towards the back of the couch. All I can see is the back of Eric's head, which doesn't tell me much. But then he turns and stares straight into me.

"You're still awake?" he asks. Fuck. Past the point of no return. I could make something up, lie to get out of it, but, no. That's not my style.

"I have to tell you something." I sit on the opposite end of the couch.

"What's wrong?" Concern appears on his face. I take a deep breath.

"A few weeks ago I dropped my lithium to 600mg."

His expression hardens. He remains silent.

"I've been feeling things that could be symptoms of mania."

He leaps off the couch.

"You did what?"

I repeat myself, sinking into the cushions. He begins to pace, shaking his head furiously.

"Why would you do that?"

"I thought it was a good idea—"

"Why would it be a good idea?"

"I thought—"

"Why would you put us at risk again?"

He doesn't want my answers. He doesn't want me to explain or defend my actions. He starts to rant about this fucking bullshit and the fucking hospital again and glares at me every time he turns around. I knew he would be upset, but I hadn't anticipated this much anger.

"I know! I'm sorry!" I say when he takes a breath.

"You think sorry is enough? You think it's okay to go batshit crazy again, to upend all of our lives again, and sorry will cover it?"

Ouch. This is the first time he's used the word crazy. Now I know he's thought it all along. No one else has said anything this cruel to describe me, at least not to my face. But for some reason, it doesn't hurt. Which is strange, because I am so sensitive that everything hurts. I don't know if he's trying to insult me, but I do know that he loves me and will always take care of me, and I don't feel offended. I guess I can recognize and admit that this is an accurate description of my manic episode last year, so there's no need to react. It's not like I'm batshit crazy all the time, or even right now. Still. Fuck.

"What symptoms are you feeling?" He practically spits out the words.

I list what I've been trying to deny: insomnia, men's attention, bright colours with halos, sensory overload, overwhelming coincidences, and too much happiness.

"How could you do this to us again? How could you be so stupid?"

Stupid. He's never called me stupid. Probably thought it many times but never said it out loud. I can accept batshit crazy. Selfish. Naïve. Gullible. Pathetic. But stupid, I am not. I made a fucking mistake. At least I'm trying to make it right before it explodes. Coming clean before I cause irreparable damage. Can't he appreciate that?

"I didn't think this would happen. I thought it would be okay." I also thought confessing was a good idea, but now I have doubts. Where is the supportive husband Dr. Patel keeps raving about? *Trust Eric.* Where is that Eric?

He stares at me, fuming and pacing. The expression on his face is the worst he's ever worn in the twenty years that I've known him.

"You need to call Dr. Patel first thing in the morning," he says.

"I know." My voice has an edge. "I came down to tell you this and that I intend to call him first thing in the morning."

"He's not going to be happy."

Obviously, but thanks. That will surely help me win tonight's battle against insomnia. Eric stops pacing and stands between me and the television, staring at me and shaking his head. I have never felt more small or alone in my life.

"I guess I'll go up," I say, standing. I turn and take a few steps. He doesn't call after me, doesn't follow me, does nothing to prevent this gap between us from growing. So much for my hope that he might help me fall asleep tonight.

"I'm a patient of Dr. Patel's. Is he there?"

The receptionist explains that he's there but unavailable, so will call me back as soon as he can. I leave my name and number and the reason why I'm calling: I'm hypomanic. He calls back within minutes.

"Charise, tell me everything—what is going on? I just saw you."

It's true, I just went for my monthly appointment, when nothing seemed amiss enough to mention. I cringe at the memory of him asking if I was taking my meds and my affirmative reply, complete with a nod and fake smile. I felt guilty then, and feel worse now.

"I know, Dr. Patel. I wasn't completely honest when you asked if I was taking my meds."

There is a pause.

"You haven't been taking your meds?" His voice sounds louder, more accusing, than a moment ago.

"I've been taking them, but a lower dose. I've been taking 600mg instead of 900mg."

A sharp inhale.

"For how long?"

"Three weeks."

A loud exhale.

"And what symptoms are you experiencing?"

I list them for him. We both know what they mean.

"Charise, I am very disappointed. Especially since you lied to me in my office."

"I know, Dr. Patel, and I am sorry. We'd talked about doing it and I was too impatient to wait. I thought it would be okay."

"It is never okay to reduce your medication on your own."

"I understand." I am close to tears. I did not expect such a scolding from my psychiatrist, or such anger from my husband. Based on their reactions, it seems like I'm the first bipolar person to ever have gone off my meds. Doesn't this happen often enough, like an addict failing after the first time in rehab, or a dieter binge-eating after a too-strict diet, that we should have discussed the possibility? Doesn't this reveal a need for better prevention or support programs for those who are newly diagnosed? Isn't this why the Alcoholics Anonymous mentor system was created? Being admonished and criticized for my mistake is not the right approach.

"This means you need to go back on olanzapine."

"No! I hate olanzapine!" The side effects of this antipsychotic drug can be brutal: weight gain, difficulty balancing, decreased sexual ability, difficulty falling or staying asleep, depression, constipation, seizures, swelling of the extremities, hives, difficulty breathing or swallowing, and unusual, involuntary repetitive face or body movements, a disorder called Tardive dyskinesia. "All I need is sleep!"

"Well, I'm sorry, but you did this to yourself, my dear."

I beg and plead with him for a few minutes until he asks for Eric. I call Eric, who immediately comes up the stairs, gives me a cold look, and takes my phone. The two of them discuss my punishment and my fate and I have no say in the matter. Just like every other woman in history who was ever declared insane. Is it any wonder we defy them by going off our meds, just to have our voices heard? I stand in the family room, clothed but feeling completely naked, awaiting my sentencing.

## 27. Good Intentions

"Guess we won't need this, eh?" I call from the mudroom. Eric sits at the other end of the house, watching a Blue Jays game with the boys. Suzie dances in front of them. She's not interested in baseball but wants to be a part of the action. Much like me.

"Hey, Eric." I walk through the kitchen flapping the letter I just received. "I guess we don't need this, right?"

He turns to look at me. He looks annoyed, maybe because I've interrupted the play, or because I still won't shut up. The olanzapine doesn't seem to be working. Neither of us want me back in the hospital but that's what will happen if it doesn't kick in soon.

I reach for a pair of scissors. I peel my brand new credit card from the letter, a replacement for the one that's about to expire, and start to cut it into small slivers.

"What are you doing?" Eric asks. He looks frustrated. I don't know why.

"We don't need it." I make the pieces smaller and smaller. Wouldn't want anyone to puzzle it back together and go on a spending spree on our dime.

Eric turns back to the game, shaking his head. Alex looks to him, then to me, then back to him. Jack's eyes haven't wavered from the television. Suzie dances on.

Am I wrong? Do I need this card? I know mine is about to expire, but I'm not supposed to overspend. Doesn't this prove I'm not manic? Why doesn't Eric see this for the goodwill gesture that it is?

"Mommy, what's for dinner?"

Dancing has worn Suzie out.

"I don't know, sweetie. Ask Daddy."

I retreat from the family room, from my family, and walk to the front of the house to lie down on a living room couch. It's not as comfortable as the family room couch, which is occupied, or our bed, which is too far away, but from here I can stare out the big windows at the magnificent trees and people passing by. So many couples always going for walks in Calgary, no matter what the weather. I want to close my eyes for a few minutes, but there are just so many interesting things to see. So many colours. It's better than a movie. Better than real life.

After a delicious Big T's BBQ dinner, I hurry the children through their bedtime routine until story time. Alex lingers in the hall outside Suzie's room, so I invite him to join the rest of us on her bed. He's too old to cuddle but he still enjoys the togetherness at the end of the day.

Once the kids are asleep, or at least pretending to be on their way to sleep, it's time to start my bedtime routine. First, kitchen cleanup. Then, a hot, soothing shower followed by yoga, herbal tea, and television. My phone has been put away for the night, but TV helps me to unwind. As long as the show is not too exciting or upsetting and I turn it off an hour before I want to fall asleep.

Eric finds me on the basement couch and we scroll through our options. Too much stimulation is a problem but it needs to be stimulating enough to hold my interest or my mind starts to wander. I suggest *Homeland*, a show we used to watch until Eric refused last summer. The last episode we saw had Claire Danes' character, who is bipolar, go off her meds to figure out who was plotting to kill her. I found it fascinating, but I guess for Eric it hit a little too close to home. Tonight we settle on an old episode of *30 Rock*, one of my favourites. It's short, and when it ends I look over at Eric to see what he wants to watch next, but he's asleep. I'm not tired yet, but I guess I should go upstairs. I drag my heels while I walk to the kitchen, pour a small amount of water into my teacup, and reach for my lithium. I hate this time of day. Hate the anxiety that starts to creep in the closer I get to switching off my bedroom light.

"Did you take your olanzapine?"

I turn. Eric stands behind me at the top of the stairs.

"I thought you were asleep," I say. I open the cap and pour three apricot-coloured pills into my hand. Eric walks towards me, reaches into the kitchen cabinet behind me, and retrieves my detested bottle of olanzapine. He hands it to me, watching so intently that I feel uncomfortable. I pry the lid off, shake a pill out, and place it in my mouth. Something tells me to hide it under my tongue, as though Eric will ask to check, but I ignore that instinct as ridiculous, and take a sip of water to wash everything down.

"Did you swallow it?" He stares at me with bloodshot eyes. Maybe my instincts aren't so ridiculous. I guess I should swallow more dramatically next time.

"Do you want to look?" I ask, in a tone that implies he'd better not. He glances at my mouth momentarily before turning away.

"Good night," I say to his retreating back. He mumbles something as he walks down the stairs but I can't make it out. Guess he's sleeping on the couch tonight. Guess I'm sleeping alone, again. Or, not sleeping, alone, again.

Now my real bedtime routine begins. The two hours leading up to this point in the night have all been about preparing my body for sleep. Now I need to prepare my mind. I head upstairs, brush my teeth, go to the bathroom, apply my salicylic acid gel to the few remaining pimples on my neck, and climb into bed. I reach for my gratitude journal. I've been writing down the happiest moments from my day for decades, since before it became a trend. Today's moments are nice: grocery shopping with Suzie, Jack decked out in his new baseball uniform for his first game, and Alex's appreciation when I offered to drive him to school so he could sleep in. Nice, low-key moments, but they make me feel good. Great, in fact.

I'm still writing when I hear the faint strum of Eric's guitar. And then his voice. Is he really playing guitar at this time of night, with the rest of the house asleep? No matter how far gone my mind is, one thing I can always rely on about my husband is that when it's bedtime, he sleeps. It's a talent I admire and am envious of. But still, it really sounds like he's playing guitar. It really sounds like he's singing. I listen, straining to hear, and sure enough, Vance Joy's words "When I see your light shine," reveal that Eric is in fact putting on a basement performance for nobody.

I slide out from under the covers and creep to the landing. But instead of getting louder, the noises go quiet. I hesitate, uncertain about whether to go downstairs or get back into bed. There are no signs from Eric, his guitar, or anything else. I go back to bed. Right after I've propped myself up on pillows and reached for *A House in the Sky* on my bedside table, the music starts again—same song, same volume. What's happening? I leave the book unopened and just sit there, listening. Maybe it's travelling up through the vents? When he starts to sing louder about the place where he wants to run, I react. I leap out of bed and scurry down the first flight of stairs and through the house until I reach the top of the basement stairs. And there I pause, for again the music has stopped. Is he intentionally playing tricks on me? Or maybe he thinks I'll yell at him for making too much noise, so he stops when he hears me? I won't be able to fall asleep without resolving this, so I silently tip-toe down the stairs to find out what's going on. And when I get there, I discover that absolutely nothing is happening. Eric is deeply asleep. His guitar sits untouched in the corner. Even the TV is off.

I tiptoe back up to bed, disoriented. I really thought I heard him. I really thought he was singing to me. I can't focus enough for my mind relaxation exercises. I reach for my phone, select the first message I see in my texts, and start to type a reply. Nothing about Eric, nothing about insomnia, just a simple greeting. A moment later, I hear a ping. I read the text. It makes me laugh. I reply. Back-and-forth this conversation goes until finally at one point the person on the other end says, "Do you know who this is?"

This snaps me back into reality. I don't know who it is. I don't have a clue. All I know is that I'm having a great time and it's far too late to be texting. I cover myself by replying "Of course," before shutting down my phone, shutting off my light, and collapsing into my bed. Not only do I not know who I was texting, I'm not even sure who *I* am.

## 28. Betrayed by the System

This room is nothing like my one last year in the psych ward ER. Or the Acute Mental Health ward as Eric calls it. Last year's room was bigger and had a raised bed, a sink, and a light switch. This year I'm in a hole. This year they're not doing an MRI, or any tests to determine if something else is wrong, because they already know I'm bipolar. This year they are not concerned. They stuck me in this hole with no water, no light switches, and a flimsy, uncomfortable excuse for a bed. And a drain in the floor. My mind doesn't want to go where it's going when I see the drain, which is the focal point of the room. I'll just have to think of a swimming pool. The floor's blue anyway, so I may as well. That's better, I like swimming pools. No, wait, I don't like swimming pools. I can barely swim.

"Hello?" I call to the people outside. Nurses and guards and doctors and maybe even Eric, I have no idea. There's no way for me to tell. The door has a window with a venetian blind but the person in the hall controls it. There's a camera mounted in the corner of this room, up high near the ceiling. It's covered with a plastic bubble. Why would it need a plastic bubble? Does it get wet? Why do they have such water issues here in a room with no water source? Could there be a reason other than the image in my head of it being hosed down, which I don't want to think about because why would it need to be hosed down? Someone said the birthing rooms are behind the locked door down the hall. Maybe if they run out they bring a birthing pool in here? But surely no woman would introduce a child into the world in this hole. I thought I was in a nice Canadian hospital. Why would it even have rooms like this? Maybe I'm in a prison instead and it's another thing they don't want to tell me.

Nobody comes to check on me so I call out again. Wave at the camera. Jump up and down to grab their attention. Nothing. The image of a birthing pool tweaked something I was supposed to remember, though.

"Where's my baby? Where's the baby?" I'm yelling now.

Still no response. I wait a second before kicking the steel door, which makes a satisfyingly loud thud despite the pain that shocks my foot. I urgently want to make that sound again, so I do. Over and over. It feels good to hear something other than my voice and the voice in my head.

"What happened to my baby? Where are my children?"

I know I sound hysterical. I am hysterical. I don't know if I'm here because I had a baby or I lost a baby or my husband wanted me locked away, but I don't think Eric wanted to get rid of me.

"Where is my husband?" I yell. Still nothing. I can't take it. I've been locked in this emergency room prison cell for what feels like days but since I have no clock and no one is answering me, I have no idea how long I've been here. Or what I'm missing on the outside. I sit at the end of the bed, the one I don't want to think of as mine even though it's in what is apparently my room. I need to rethink my strategy. They don't open the door when I yell, so maybe they would listen to a polite request. I stand again.

"Hello?" I call out hopefully and then rap against the window three times. "Can I use the bathroom, please?"

Nothing.

"Hello?" I try again. "I really need the bathroom." I really do. I'm not a liar, even if I hallucinate and sometimes hear things when I'm manic, I still don't say anything that I know to be untrue.

There is no response. I sit calmly on the bed. I can show them that I'm reasonable and can wait. I just wish I knew who was testing me in here. The security guards? Peace officers? Doctors? Nurses? Who are my tormentors outside that door making the decision to ignore my pleas for help?

A little bit longer turns into a lot longer—too much longer. Somewhere out there, wherever out there is, I have a family and a husband who won't let me rot to death in this hole. I look at their framed picture and am overwhelmed with love. Sitting beside the frame on the bed, because I am not privileged enough to have a bedside table, is the plastic bag with chocolate that Eric packed for me. I would love to eat it, but my patience ran out long ago and anger is taking over. I stand, walk the few steps to the steel door with its faux window, and bang my fist against the reinforced glass so hard that the pain reverberates up my arm.

"Hey. You. Whoever is there. Anyone. I need the bathroom."

A gruff man in a security guard's uniform fiddles with the blinds and they open for a second, just long enough for him to scowl and say, "No," before he snaps them closed again.

This time I crumple. Not to the floor, because even though it's blue and I love blue, that drain is taunting me. Besides, floors are dirty, and this ER one is fucking disgusting. My shoulders sag, my spine curves, and I collapse onto the edge of my bed, dejected and unsure about what to do. What more could I possibly do? I'm talking to myself but I'm also talking out loud, which doesn't matter since no one's listening anyway, and my warbly voice is getting carried away with emotion. Carried away with tears, moans, and wails. I force myself to take a deep breath, calm down, and not give them the satisfaction of seeing that they've broken me. After a few exhalations, it's time for a different strategy: rage.

I stand up, shoulders back, and start to pound the window with my fist. When that elicits no reaction, I kick the bottom while punching the top. When that still elicits no reaction, I back up to take a running start and bash my head into the steel door. Repeatedly. Finally, I'm too dizzy to stand so I drop to the floor. I'm sitting, propped up on one arm, but soon enough that arm gives out and I'm lying in this disgusting swimming pool and I can't do anything about it. After staring at the filth long enough to regain some energy, I push myself up to crawl to the bed. I climb up and curl into the fetal position, so worn out and in such shock that I don't even cry.

I stay this way for a long time. Maybe an hour passes, maybe a day, I have no way of knowing. Nobody checks on me, brings me food, or offers to help me in any way. At some point, I pull myself up from this flimsy mattress that has God knows what stains soaked into it, squat to pee into the swimming pool drain, and begin to pace. Not in straight lines, but in circles, around the drain. I need to accept this drain for what it is, so it loses its power over me. Time passes. I keep walking, numb. I don't know what else to do. There is nothing else I can do. My mind slowly starts to wake up again and with it, the anger. The anger is telling me how unfair this treatment is, how inhumane for hospital staff to do this to a mentally ill patient, or any patient. My anger tells me to do something—not to sit back and let them treat me like this. But what? Calm and polite didn't work. Rage only left me with a headache and bruises. Then I spy the magazines Eric packed. House and Home, Style at Home, People, Us. Why did he think I wanted these? They're so clean. So perfect. So stupid. Yeah, I can use those.

I sit on the edge of the bed again. I go through each magazine methodically, ripping page after page into the tiniest confetti I can create. I take pleasure in watching a pile of snowflakes build up at my feet. This is the first thing I've done here that feels like creative expression. When I'm almost finished making it snow in this seasonless room, I finally, hear the noise I'd forgotten I was listening for: the click of the lock on my door. I look up to see the door swing open as if it was the most natural thing in the world, and a woman walk in as if she owned the place. She is one of them. A security guard. Or peace officer. Or whatever it is they are. She introduces herself while towering above me. She looks tough. She looks like a tough motherfucking bitch. She wouldn't have time for me in real life. A guard man follows her. He shakes his head and clucks as he takes what is left of my magazines and a few clumps of snow and puts them into a garbage bag. He surveys the room, shakes his head again, scowls at me, and leaves. I want to call out after him, demanding that he return those items, even the snow, because they're mine. But I bite my tongue. If he comes back, he'll confiscate my framed picture, hidden by their flimsy excuse for a pillow. I've lost everything else; I can't lose that too. It's the only evidence that my family is real.

"May I sit on your bed?" the woman says, as though I have a say in anything she does. I gesture to the space beside me. There is obviously nowhere else for her to sit since my room contains nothing else other than a drain.

"They've asked me to talk to you to find out why you're so upset. To see how we can help."

I stare at her. The men have sent in this woman, who is one of them but also one of us, because they are too chicken shit to send in one of their own. One of their own who's actually causing the problem by locking me in here. Another woman cleaning up another man's mess. No matter what we do in this world, they will only ever see us as their cleaning ladies. Their whores.

"I was told you were ramming your head against the door."

I nod. It was ages ago. No one bothered to check for a head, foot, or hand injury. Only the best healthcare here in this mental health ER. Or Acute Mental Health ward. Or Acute Inpatient Unit. Or whatever the fuck it's called.

"I asked them to open it and they wouldn't," I say. My words are tentative, probing. I don't trust this woman. She feels like a threat. She is dressed in an intimidating costume and acts tough to be intimidating. They sent me a threat wrapped in a woman's body to lull me into a false sense of security. Or peace. Or protection. Or whatever they call it. They should have sent the nice one who accompanied me from the ER up to the ward last year. She was butchier than this one, who is all angles and sinew, but she had smiling eyes. This one's face is cold. Hard. She's not even pretending to smile.

She asks further and I explain further. The more I talk, the more I open up, even though there is a wall between us. I tell her that there's no air in here and I feel like I'm suffocating. That they wouldn't let me out to use the bathroom. That I feel like a prisoner, or a princess locked in a tower. At some point I move from my spot beside her to kneel on the floor at her feet. Like a beggar. With no dignity. Because that's what I am now. That's what they've made me.

"All I want is for the door to be open. If the door is open I'll be quiet. I won't yell, I won't go into the hall, I just need the door open."

My hands are folded together as though in prayer. As though I am praying to her. She nods her head, looks like she's considering my request, and then stands, casting me aside.

"I'll see what I can do."

She leaves, and I watch her walk away with the expectation that she'll return to let me know the decision of the men who hold the power. Less than a minute later the door is slammed shut, the lock clicks into place, and the overhead light I have no control over is switched off. And I don't know if I'll ever get out of here again. That fucking bitch. I knew she was one of them.

## 29. The Long Weekend

"What's your name?" I say from the confines of my hole. We've reached a compromise: the door can be open if I stay in my prison cell and don't get rowdy. It was my nurse who told me this good news when he came in to check my vitals. I don't know how we got here after last night's betrayal, or this morning's betrayal, or yesterday's betrayal, or whenever it was that I was betrayed, but somehow we're here. All good. Pretending nothing happened. Pretending I never used the drain as a toilet. I think it was the shift change. The tired staff went home when these fresh guys came in and they have more patience for me. This guard doesn't mind if I talk to him from the doorway. He keeps responding and hasn't told me to be quiet, plus he's laughing at my jokes. I make a lot of jokes when I'm manic. It was the same last time I was here, exactly one year ago. I am very funny and entertaining when I'm not furious or seductive.

"Liam," he says, glancing quickly at me with a smile before returning to his monitor.

"Nice to meet you, Liam, I'm Charise." He nods. Of course he already knows my name, but introducing myself feels civilized. He must have looked at my file. Or am I being grandiose? Is it arrogant to think this security guy knows my name because he has access to my records? Am I flattering myself, thinking everybody is attracted to me, becoming hypersexual? Oh, shit, what was his name? I've forgotten. I can't ask him again or he'll think I'm crazy. Hah.

"You know I'm bipolar, right?"

He doesn't answer. One thing that's different about this trip compared to last year is that everybody already knows I'm bipolar. Last year they were still trying to figure it out, with their tests and compassion. This year they have the diagnosis, blame me for fucking with my meds, and don't pretend to care. Bipolar is a one-size-fits-all label in their eyes. In their eyes, it's my fault I'm here. It's all my fault.

"Where are you from?" I say, trying a different approach to figure out his name.

"Right here." He smiles. His dark hair looks long enough to fall in his eyes, but he slicks it back so it stays helmet-like atop his head. I watch for a strand to escape but, like me, it can't. This guy in charge of mental ER security is just so young. Just so cute. He knows it too. He knows how to use his smile for full effect.

"As in Calgary? You were born here?"

He nods. I wish I knew his name.

"Funny. I would have thought you were Spanish or Irish or something."

He gives me a look.

"Those are very different," he says. There's that smile again.

"I know. You know what I mean though."

He laughs. I don't think he knows what I mean. I don't know exactly what I mean. He looks Spanish but something about him says Irish. I don't know what. What was his name again?

"There's something about you that seems Irish. I'm part Irish," I say. He starts talking about his background and I try to listen but I can't focus. It's not because he's dreamy, although he is, but because I need to know his name. What would non-manic me do in this situation? Maybe ask again? That would be okay if I wasn't on my way to the Psych ward. Society rules are different here. I can't show weakness because that's what they're preying on.

"Have you seen *The LEGO Movie*?" I say. He gives me a quizzical look. I must have interrupted him.

"Sorry," I say. "It's just, there are these cops in that movie and you remind me of them." Maybe. I'm not sure if I remember the movie properly.

"I can't say I've seen it," he says. Another smile.

"Do you have kids?"

He chuckles. Shakes his head.

"Well, when you have kids watch it with them. You'll see what I mean. You're just like the LEGO guy."

"If you say so." His eyes twinkle.

I am no closer to figuring out this man's name, so I have to do the next best thing.

"Is it okay if I give you a nickname?" I say.

He gives me a peculiar look, as though I'm the first patient to ever ask such a thing.

"What nickname?"

"I was thinking Irish. But now, maybe, LEGO guy?"

He starts to laugh.

"Is it okay?" I say. He doesn't look offended but I want to be sure. If there is one thing I do not want to do it's offend the warden.

"Sure. I can't say I've ever had either of those for a nickname before," he says. There's that smile again. If only we weren't in a hospital and I was a decade or two younger. And single.

"Okay, so if I say it you'll know I'm just being friendly, right?"

"Okay," he says, still wearing that smile. Looks like I figured out his name after all.

"Can I walk down the hall?" I say. I've been so calm lately that they've started letting me have fresh air. If hospital hallway air can be considered fresh. Aren't prisoners given yard time or something for real fresh air? What I wouldn't give for that right now.

"In a bit," he says. "Just wait until your nurse comes back."

"Okay, thanks." This time I smile. I have a good smile. Powerful. He hesitates a moment before turning to his computer. From the look on his face, he'd like it if we weren't in a hospital too. Doesn't look like he cares that I'm forty-one and married.

I sit up on the bed, groggy. For some reason the door is closed even though I remember it being open the last time I checked. Seeing it shut makes me nervous. I start to breathe deeply to maintain some control. I look up at the ceiling and focus on the image in my head of Eric bringing me here. I can see him driving up, getting out to open my door, and walking me into the hospital entrance. I asked what we were doing, because the sight of the hospital stressed me out even though I've been coming as an out-patient for a year without incident. He replied, "We're making a play." This is how I know it didn't happen. It is so unlike him, all of it. He never opens my door. Would never make a play. It doesn't make sense. Have I been asleep? Did I fall asleep waiting for my nurse to let me out to roam the halls? Well, the hall. There is only one hall. It makes an L-shape past the nurse's station, leading to the kitchen and a locked door. But still, better than this cage. Back to the point, how could I have fallen asleep? That is so unlike me.

I am still on the bed trying to figure out if I was dreaming and also trying to figure out what the stains are on the ceiling when I hear a knock on the door and it swings open. Eric walks in, wearing a tentative smile and holding a piece of paper.

"Hi, Reesie, how are you feeling?" He sits beside me.

"Fuzzy. What happened when you dropped me off ?"

"What?"

"What happened when you brought me here?" I don't want to tell him what I remember, which must have been a dream, because he will really think I'm crazy. It just seemed so real. I still feel his breath on my ear when he whispered those words.

"Okay, I'll tell you. But first, do you remember that form from last year?"

I give him a look. Don't start with that fucking form.

"She had trouble with this last year too," he says, turning to his right. Only then do I notice that someone else, someone official, is here too. It's a man and I think he's wearing a nurse's uniform but he looks blurry. I feel so foggy. How long has he been here?

"Reese, you have to sign this form. The same one as last year about being an involuntary patient."

Something hits me and I start to laugh. This is so ridiculous.

"Oh, okay, Eric," I say in a purposely condescending tone. "Where's the form?" He puts the paper in front of me and hands me a pen. "Look at me, here I am, voluntarily signing a form that says I'm involuntary. It's one of the stupidest things ever but you're the lawyer and I must obey." I cap the pen and start to spin it on my fingers. Eric hands the form to the nurse, who says something too quiet for my ears. Eric takes the pen and hands it to the coward, who leaves the room. Eric looks relieved.

I want to ask him about that man and when he walked into the room, but I don't want to let on that I don't know. Things are happening to me without my knowledge or permission but if I ask questions it'll make it worse.

"When we got here we drove to the underground parking and while I was trying to park you started getting upset so you undid your seatbelt and jumped out."

Right. I kind of remember that. A little.

"What was I upset about?"

"You kept talking about the baby. The pregnancy."

"What baby?" I say.

Eric looks at me long and hard. Trying to decide how much to tell me and what my feeble mind can handle.

"You thought you were pregnant and the baby died."

From the look on his face there is more, but that's all he'll say. He's a vault when he wants to be.

"Huh. That's not how I remembered it." I like my dream version better. I wish he had told me we were making a play. I would love to make a play.

"Do you remember when we were in triage and you broke the nurse's door?"

I guess he's decided my mind is not too fragile for this information.

"What nurse?"

"The one who was assessing you. You got up and pulled at her door until you broke it."

"Oh. The one who was Chad last year."

"What?" Eric's face reveals pure confusion.

"Chad was the guy who did that assessment last year. The one I kept saying wasn't good at his job and needed acting classes."

"Right. That guy."

"Anyway, I didn't break her door. It was a sliding door that was blocked; I just lifted it and knocked it off its track."

"No, you broke it." I think he's being dramatic, but he's the sane one so I'm supposed to accept whatever version of events he tells me. I have to start being compliant again, no matter what. I look down so he won't see me roll my eyes. If I argue then I am argumentative, yet another symptom of mania, so rolling my eyes secretly is currently the only option I have. I could fix that door in less than a minute.

"How are the kids?" I say to change the subject, and also because I desperately need to know.

"They're great. They're really great kids." He pulls out his phone to show me pictures of just how great they are and how much fun they're having without me, which makes me miss them terribly. I feel tears, but I don't want to cry because again, displaying emotions is only acceptable for normal non-mentally ill people. This cramped room feels even more claustrophobic with Eric here.

"I guess you should get back to them," I say. My voice sounds short and tight. "Give them hugs for me."

Eric looks at me like there's something more to say, stands, and pulls me into his arms. He leans down and squeezes me tightly. I keep my feet flat on the floor, not going up on tip-toes like I usually do to bridge the height difference between us, and wrap my arms loosely around his neck. It is an expressive hug, but it doesn't express what he wants it to express because he's not saying the things I want him to say.

"What time is it?" I say, as I walk Eric to the door.

"Morning. Around ten."

I look to the desk and notice a different security guard in Irish LEGO guy's place. I wonder what time we were talking. Did I somehow sleep through the night after our conversation? It seems unlikely.

"Morning," I say to the new guy. He's even younger than Irish guy. He doesn't hear me, or pretends not to, and continues his work.

"I'll be back soon, okay?" Eric says. I nod. Soon is a relative concept. Especially when I have no clock.

"Okay, Charise, you can walk to the kitchen and back, but you have to be quiet."

Jay looks at me with pleading eyes. I don't know why he's so desperate. I remember Jay from last time. He was kind then, just like he's been kind now. He was real. Not vague and not false. Genuine. I told him I remembered him and his kindness when he re-introduced himself to me yesterday. Or whenever it was.

"Okay," I say, smiling as though being quiet won't be a problem. I take a few steps before turning back.

"Jay," I say in a hushed voice. He looks at me with mild exasperation. "Is it okay if I get a popsicle?"

He nods and waves me away. I'm not sure how I know about the popsicles but somehow I do. Pleased with myself, I walk straight to the kitchen and open the freezer door. I choose a red one. I like red. I sit at the table to enjoy this treat without the distraction of walking or people. When I finish, I stand and start to slowly walk back. I don't want the hole.

I pass an open door and my head automatically swivels to glance inside. A young woman sits on her bed, staring at me. I stop and rest against her doorframe. I know I'm not allowed to cross the threshold; that was one of the rules from last year.

"Hi," I say.

She nods and gives me a bleak smile.

"Charise, you can't go in patients' rooms." Jay's voice travels across the nurse's desk.

"I'm not," I say. There is some defiance in my voice, but I give Jay an innocent, playful smile. People always fall for my smile. But not Jay. He gives me a look, so I start to walk. It's too bad. That woman seemed just as bored and lonely as I am.

At the corner of the nurse's station, where the hall to the kitchen meets the hall to my room, I notice an interesting looking printer sitting close to the edge of the desk. I stop to investigate. It's a barcode printer, something I used to code to interact with our robots, but compared to the ones I worked with it looks futuristic.

"Do you need something? Are you in pain?" A nurse I don't recognize rolls her chair towards me. She looks concerned. I guess nobody's told her that I've already been diagnosed.

"No, thanks. I'm just looking at your printer. I used to work with similar equipment when I was a robotics engineer. They were tricky to program, but I figured it out." I tap my forehead and smile at her, happy with our interaction and the memories of my old job. As I reflect upon my good old days, I notice a security guard, another new one but this guy's older, shake his head and roll his eyes. He's a few feet away from me, so I look around to see what might be causing his dismissive, disrespectful body language. But there is nothing. Is he reacting because of me? Because of my interest in the barcode printer? My career building robots?

"Is something funny?" I ask, genuinely curious. I would love a laugh. He scowls and stares at the floor.

"Back to your room," he says in a gruff voice.

I take another step. And another. And another. But I'm slowing down. My eye catches an interesting display on the opposite wall, behind the nurse's station. There are three horizontal pipes with valves, locked behind a glass access door like a fire extinguisher. From my vantage point and with the dim lighting in that corner, it looks terribly artistic. So industrial yet so pleasing to the eye. Someone put a lot of thought into the aesthetics of this practical necessity. I'm impressed.

As I stare at the wall, I notice yet another security guard. They all look so similar in their greige uniforms. This one stands beside the valves, and I think he thinks I'm staring at him, because he swivels his head and moves around as though I've put him under a microscope. He then fixes me with a hard glare.

"Sorry," I say. "I'm just admiring the display. Doesn't it look like they've been framed and hung in an art gallery?"

The guy looks, then looks back at me, and then takes a step to his left. Blocking my view of the valves. Okay, then.

"Charise, it's time to go back in your room. We can leave your door open if you're quiet." Jay is suddenly beside me, as though I need a personal escort.

I nod and take a step towards the door. But I cannot do it.

"Please, Jay, can I stand in the hall? Please? I'll be quiet. I'll stand right here." I move beside the door and face the nurses' station, because I can't even bear to look in the hole. Jay glances away and I turn my head to follow his gaze, but I'm too late. I don't know what the security guard said in the moment their eyes locked, but I can guess.

"Sorry, Charise, but no," Jay says.

He moves to accompany me into the room. I can tell he doesn't want to.

"How about here then?" I say, pleading with him as I step onto the threshold's blue tile where it meets the hallway's grey tile. "Can I stand here?"

Jay shakes his head again after looking at the guard.

"Here?" I take a step further, my volume increasing as my frustration mounts. "Here. I'll drown in your swimming pool, how about that?"

Jay sighs.

"Okay, now we have to close the door. Can you go in all the way please?"

"No!" I yell. "He keeps barricading me with invisible walls that are really glass ceilings. Next he'll say I'm a nasty woman!"

No one reacts. They're too bored to feel sympathetic or try to understand. My words make perfect sense to me, but I'm the only one curious and concerned enough to think them through. These overworked people, whether kind and gentle or hostile and rough, are tired. They've seen it all in the ER psych ward. They're just waiting for their shifts to end.

I start to scream and resist but the next thing I know, I'm back in the hole. I don't know if it was Jay or a guard who manhandled me in, but somebody must have. I didn't walk in on my own. I guess I'm officially involuntary after all.

"You stupid fucking asshole! Don't you fucking lock me in here again. LEGO guy I fucking hate you! Do you know who I am? Do you know who my husband is? You are so fucking fired, you have no idea what we can do." These threats are surprising, even to me. And then they're hilarious. I pause to look at the security camera on my left, close to the ceiling. An image appears in the plastic shield's reflection. It's fuzzy at first, but I blink and it starts to focus. It's Eric, relaxing on our basement couch, eating a bowl of popcorn one kernel at a time, like he's watching a movie. I'm the movie. Or the play. I do a double-take to try to make sense of this, and as I stare at him, he sees me, waves, and gives me a big thumbs up. I am stunned into silence. Is this real? Did Eric somehow put some kind of two-way video wiretap on the shield to keep tabs on me from home? He is tall enough.

But, surely not. Could this be a hallucination? From whatever drug cocktail they're giving me or from sleep deprivation? Or a psychotic delusion? If it is a figment of my overactive imagination, is it because I'm bipolar or because my mind knows I need something hopeful, protection to survive this trauma, an escape from my current reality? Like Amanda Lindhout dissociating from her body while being raped. I don't understand how I see Eric so clearly, like we're FaceTiming with holograms. I'll have to think it through. Right now, it doesn't matter. His broad smile and that simple thumbs-up are all the motivation I need to keep yelling, keep slamming my head into the door, and keep doing what I'm doing. Sooner or later, they'll have to let me out. Sooner or later, Eric will rescue me. The prince always rescues the princess.

Hours have passed. Days, maybe. I don't know what time it is, but I know I'm awake and I'm not supposed to be. I also know it is the middle of the night, because I've been here long enough to figure out their routines. This room is dark, because they control when I have night or day in here, but the hall is dark too. The gap at the edges between the venetian blinds inside the door's window and the steel window frame allows some hallway light to pass through. Leonard Cohen was right—*there is a crack in everything*. This small amount of light is all I have to soothe me right now, so I can't let them know or they would take it away. Right now, it is dim, and the halls are quiet. No visitors, no new patients, a skeleton staff. Night.

I must have slept for a while, because I can't remember the last time I ate. Or the last time I saw my children. I picture their faces, and rub my fingers along the frame of our family photograph underneath my pillow, but it makes me so sad that tears spring fresh and I have to stand up. I have to distract myself or the sadness will swallow me whole, deep in the belly of this whale's swimming pool. I don't even know what I'm stuck in anymore.

Not enough energy to pace, so I go and stand beside my door. Try to peek through the gap to see what's going on. A nurse is doing something behind the desk. Something on the computer. I doubt it's work. I remember him from last year. He was sleazy. There's a guard I don't recognize standing almost out of my view. He looks like he's doing nothing other than staring at a column.

I don't want them to see me, I want to stay a fly on the wall, but I realize now why I woke up. I need the bathroom. Dread fills me because I know they're not going to be happy.

"Hello?" I call out as I gently knock on the door. I see the nurse's head turn. "May I use the bathroom please?"

The sleazy nurse sighs and I see him roll his eyes. The guard doesn't flinch. They both ignore me and keep doing whatever it is they're doing. Whatever it is that's more important than tending to a patient in their hospital who needs their help.

"Hello?" I try again. I know it's futile. But this is worse than last time. This is not just pee. "I really need to go."

Nothing. I try and I try, my voice wavering and my knocking becoming more desperate. I explain why, embarrassed, but I have no dignity left and they need to know the urgency of the situation. I can't do that in here. I don't have water or soap. I don't even have toilet paper. They took away my magazines. No response. They don't care. At all.

It's too late, I can't stop it. I hike up this awful gown and squat over the drain. I close my eyes, even though I can barely see anyway. I force myself to remember playing volleyball on the beach in Ixtapa only four months ago. How has my life gone so horribly wrong in only four months? I picture the boys burying Suzie in the sand, a huge grin on her face, and the kids delighting in their virgin drinks at the kids-only bar. I force myself to deny the reality of my current situation, because this can't truly be my life right now. This is just wrong.

I have nothing to clean myself with, nothing to wash my hands. Nothing. I collapse onto the awful bed, saddened by the realization that I am now just as filthy, if not filthier, than this mattress. Than this room. This is where I belong. Silent tears come, and I don't fight them. I don't resist, I don't embrace. I just lie there, curled in the fetal position. Defeated. Tears filling the mattress.

I wake from a deep sleep when I hear the lock click. I open my eyes, afraid of who is about to enter and what is about to happen. A head appears and I pull my knees tightly to my chest. It's sleaze nurse. I'm terrified, but I'm also so fucking tired that I can't sit, scream, or do anything other than hug myself and try to hold onto any last threads of sanity I still possess. There can't be many.

"Time to check your vitals," he says too cheerfully, wheeling in that machine they use to test my blood or pulse or whatever the fuck they pretend to care about.

"Now?" I say with a thick, dry croak. I can't remember the last time I had water.

"Oh, is that a turd?" he says, as though it's a surprise discovery and also not surprising at all. As though I didn't tell him it was about to happen what, two, three hours ago? As though the surveillance camera in my room "for my protection" didn't confirm that I was doing exactly what I said I had to do. As though he really came in here, in the middle of what is still night based on the darkness in the hall, to check my vitals. As though THAT is vital enough to wake a manic patient when she's finally deeply asleep, for once.

I say nothing. He picks up my shit with a gloved hand as though he does this all the time. Maybe he does. Which is dreadful. He does whatever he claims he needs to do with that stupid machine, gives me another fucking pill to make me more confused, and leaves. I close my eyes. For once I am relieved to hear the lock click and be left alone, in my flimsy gown with nowhere to hide. I have no idea what that man is capable of and I've read too many true stories about similar situations. Similar assholes who long ago stopped seeing patients as people and started seeing them as opportunities.

The darkness is too bright outside my closed eyelids. I feel someone pulling at my arm before I hear a voice.

"Come on, we've got to clean you up."

This voice sounds familiar, but they all sound the same now, and the familiar ones are starting to be unrecognizable, so I don't know who this is. My eyes are just as groggy as my ears, but I force them open. Everything is a blur. The only things I can distinguish are blobs of colour and darkness and light. My eyelids instinctively close. I am too broken to feel afraid. My whole body is asleep but I try to comply. I'm still trying to hold onto hope and I know that compliance is the only good way out of this place. They taught me well last year. My legs are just so heavy. They've never felt this heavy before.

My arm is wrapped around somebody's shoulder and I am half-carried, half-dragged out of the room. I don't see this happen because my eyes refuse to stay open, but I feel the rush of fresh stale hospital corridor air when we walk through the doorway. I'm taken somewhere, I don't know, and someone adjusts my gown. I think I'm sitting. Then I feel water. I haven't felt water in so long. It is more soothing than I could have imagined.

"Is it too hot?"

I open my eyes. I think it's Eric, staring into me with concern. I blink in slow-motion. He's doing something with his hands and bubbles, but I think it's him. I'm not sure. I think it is. I don't know. It's too much. It's just too much. I'm drowning.

# 30. Beaten Down

Where are we going? I have no idea but I'm relieved to be going somewhere. Anywhere away from this room. It feels good to be leaving. I must have finally slept well to feel so good. So light and clear. This morning's yoga helped too. With nothing else to do, I began my familiar routine on the flimsy mattress as a fuck-you, to show them I am capable of making healthy choices to control my emotions. It was also a healthy choice to control my emotions. The guards and nurses must have been surprised to see my switch from rage to zen. I bet they got a kick out of my cow pose in this flimsy gown. I bet they got a real kick out of that.

I step away from the door that has confined me for an eternity to follow the young, cute security guard down the hall. Or is he a peace officer? Someone explained the difference to me back when we were on friendlier terms, but I forget. Their uniforms are so similar.

Are they transferring me to a room? Did they find a bed? Is this a supervised visit to the bathroom because they don't want a repeat of what happened the last time? I'd ask Irish LEGO guy but he seems pissed. Maybe he's not having a good day. Maybe he didn't sleep well. I know how that feels.

He might have told me where we're going, just like he once told me his name and I promptly forgot. I don't think so though. I think he barked a terse "Come with me," after unlocking my door. It seems that cute LEGO guy has now turned into surly LEGO guy. Which makes him even more like Bad Cop/Good Cop from the movie. I squeeze my lips to stifle a smile. I think if he notices that I'm amused it'll make things worse.

I wonder if I did something. It'd be nice if he joked again. I know I've been yelling for them to let me out of that room. That dark, dirty, claustrophobic, airless, haunted, motherfucking room. Maybe I said something he didn't like. It wouldn't surprise me. According to these people, I have anger and trust issues because I don't believe strangers who pretend to be friends. Pretend to know everything about me when they don't know me at all. Wouldn't anyone being held prisoner, trapped in a cage, with no light, no water, and no end in sight, have anger issues? Maybe LEGO guy's mad because I didn't pay him enough positive attention. He realized I'm not entirely under his thumb. I remember him scolding me for going into rooms even though I wasn't. I was in the hall, introducing myself to other lonely, bored, desperate crazy people, who were happy to see me. I know it's forbidden to cross the threshold, even if the patient gives permission. I'm trying to be compliant.

We are only a few steps down the hall when it occurs to me that I might not come back. They might be transferring me to the ward, finally. This makes me so excited that I clasp my hands together and pause momentarily. And then I realize that my only prized possession is still back in that room. That fucking room. I don't want to go back, I really don't want to go back, but I can't leave my family behind. I can't trap them in the hole too.

"Oh! I forgot something. I'll just grab it," I say.

I turn, quickly take a few steps, and dash back into the room. The place I've been trying to escape for forever. My spirits plummet, so I tell myself to hurry up, get the picture, and get out. The vibe in this room is so bad. This is a place where dark things happen. I cross the room and lift the framed picture from underneath my pillow, feeling immediately calmed by the sight of my loving family. I see movement out of the corner of my eye and turn to see LEGO guy approaching. He doesn't look happy.

"I got it," I say with excitement, lifting the frame to show him my pride and joy. "Now we can go."

But he grabs me, knocking it from my hand, and spins me around to face the corner, locking both hands in his, behind my back. I hear the thin, delicate frame break when my picture hits the concrete swimming pool floor, and I start to cry. I can't believe he did that to my family. My tears make it worse. He is on me like a bouncer tossing a drunk to the curb. He twists my left arm to pin my hand to the back of my head while still holding my right hand behind my back. Then he forces me onto my sorry excuse for a bed, face first. Not satisfied with this level of containment he jams his knee into my groin, resulting in an explosion of pain, while I struggle to turn my head so I can breathe. I yell and gasp for air as another peace officer, or security guard, rushes into this godforsaken room. To distract me through this moment where things are moving too quickly yet time seems to be stopped, I focus on trying to figure out which one is peace and which one is security. I think the older one might be here to help me, but I'm not sure. Maybe he wants in on the fun. There is a second knee to my groin before LEGO guy releases me. The older guy must have pulled him off because I saw the look in his eyes. He wasn't planning to stop.

"I'm just getting my picture." I sob, standing as soon as the pressure of his body is gone. I know they'll say this is defiance, and it might encourage them to throw me down again, but I have to get up. He can't think he won. "You didn't have to do that!" I cry and yell incoherently. I look at my broken photograph on the floor. Now it's tainted with ugliness, just like everything else in here. "I couldn't leave without my family."

They both stare at me and step back, away from the angry, unstable mental patient. Irish is forcing himself to breathe. His eyes are huge, fists clenched, and mouth forms an aggressive sneer. He looks like he wants to pound on me and would be doing so if it weren't for the older guy. He's not sorry. The older guy looks nervous, and at first I think it's because he realizes that his younger colleague lost control and made a mistake, which could cause problems for them. But then I wonder if that's not the reason. If it's because he seriously believes that I could be dangerous. As though my petite body is a threat to a lumberjack and a gym rat. Their combined weight has to be triple mine. Does he not see this? Is he so incapable of logic, of rational thought, that he can't distinguish between what is literally standing in front of him and what he has been told about bipolar people? Does he think being manic gives me superhuman strength?

"Why did you do that?" I say. "Why do you have to be so cruel? How do you think I'll react when you keep treating me like an animal? How am I supposed to break this cycle alone?"

They mutter to each other but offer no consolation or explanation. My body is shaking, so before my knees give out I collapse onto the bed, holding my head in my hands. The pain in my groin explodes the moment I sit, which forces me to clench my pelvis and distracts me enough to stop crying. The sudden silence is stifling, and it makes me realize that they're gone. I've been left alone. I look up to confirm what I already know: the door is closed. I've been locked in this room, again. I lie on my side in the fetal position to alleviate the fire below. I should have known I wasn't going anywhere. I should have known I can't trust anyone.

# 31. Losing Everything

"I'm sorry, what's your name again?"

"Janine." She smiles. I'm so glad I've finally been transferred to the Mental Health unit. The staff are much more patient and kind.

"Janine. Sorry. I keep forgetting names." I keep forgetting a lot. I don't know what drugs they gave me in the ER but whatever I'm coming down from is bad. Worse than last year. It frustrates me that I can't remember Janine's name. She has shown so much compassion. She's never suggested my illness is a threat. That what I do remember is a delusion.

"It's okay," she says kindly. "You have a lot to remember."

"Yes," I nod. "What time is breakfast again?"

"Eight o'clock."

I look at the digital clock on the wall. It's seven-twelve. Below the clock is a sign that reads, 'Today is Wednesday.' I don't think it's Wednesday. It doesn't feel like a Wednesday. But I don't know. For all I know it's not even 2018 anymore.

"Could I make tea, please?" I don't remember much but I remember how to make tea. Even in a psych ward. Last year, tea and coffee were stored in the kitchen, and patients could help themselves. Now, they're behind the desk and we need to ask, so they can monitor our caffeine. I'm impressed by this change. I like that they're trying to improve. Manic patients should not have a lot of caffeine, but we crave instant gratification and have little to no self-control. Hopefully they'll rethink the meals in here too. Less carbs and sugar, and more fresh produce, improve anyone's mental stability.

Janine asks for my preference and hands me an Earl Grey tea bag. I'm about to leave when I remember something else.

"Sorry, Janine. What time will Eric come today?" My voice falters. I don't know if she'll say nine a.m. or five p.m. because I don't know what day it is. My mind can't process the difference between weekday and weekend visiting hours since every day feels the same and also because other people visit whenever they want, no matter what day it is. Nobody else seems to stick to visiting hours, just like last year. Sometimes it feels like the nurses are testing us, to see how obedient we are, just like last year. It also feels like they only enforce certain rules with me. Like I'm the black sheep or they just enjoy playing good-cop-bad-cop for fun. Just like last year.

"Do you want to call and ask him?"

I pause to consider this.

"Am I allowed to use the phone this early?"

She nods. So it wasn't a test or it was and I passed.

"Okay, that's a good idea."

She hands me the cordless phone but keeps holding on even after I've reached to take it out of her hand. I look into her eyes.

"I'm sure he'll be here as soon as he can. He did say yesterday that he had to get some work done before he could come."

"He did? Yesterday?" I don't remember that at all. "What day is it?"

"Tuesday."

Tuesday. So, not Wednesday. But I came here on Friday. I think.

"I came to the hospital on Friday, right Janine?"

She nods.

"The Friday before Mother's Day."

She nods again.

"So I missed Mother's Day." I exhale the breath I didn't realize I'd been holding. Janine puts one hand over top of mine on the phone.

"And I missed my mom's birthday."

She smiles a sad smile.

"Try to give your husband a call, Charise. He'll be happy to hear your voice."

I don't know if he'll be happy to hear my voice. Ever since I told him about the security guard he seems afraid of what I might reveal next. But I want to know if he filed the complaint, like he said he would. And I want to hear his voice.

Janine lets go of the phone. I stare at the buttons, too numb to cry.

"I don't know his number." My phone remembers it for me. Janine takes the phone, glances at my file to retrieve Eric's contact information, and starts to dial. I rub the top of my head, still bruised from slamming it into the ER steel door, not my most clever idea. I can't bring myself to touch the back of my head, bruised from that asshole pinning me down, because it feels too raw. I'm trying to avoid that memory, even though I know I have to recall every detail to hold him accountable. To hold the hospital accountable. To train their staff better. To prevent this kind of abuse. But I tried to sit on the exercise bike yesterday, something that helped me last year in the psych ward, and my groin hurt so badly I had to climb off. It's going to hurt for days. It also burns when I pee. I wonder if he could have caused a urinary tract infection. Jesus. I came to the hospital for mental problems and I'll leave with a broken body. No wonder I have trust issues. According to Dr. Patel, my paranoia and inability to trust him the moment we met was a symptom of being bipolar. I'm sure he's still making the same assessment for anyone admitted to the ER who doesn't fully believe him, a stranger, upon being introduced.

"It's ringing." Janine hands me the phone. I nod my thanks and walk away, anxious for Eric to pick up and hoping I don't wake him or our children. It is such a relief to hear the click of connection and then his voice say hello. I sit in one of the comfy chairs near the window and look up through the glass at the glorious sky. I take a deep breath, remind myself that I'm not in that room anymore, the security guards can't hurt me here, and I'm one day closer to going home.

"Hi Eric," I say. "Did I wake you?"

"Janine, could I have a Band-Aid please?" I prop my leg on a chair to show her the cut on my ankle, and speak loudly for the nearby security guards to hear. "I cut myself shaving. I just keep getting wounded in this hospital."

I don't know why there are so many guards lurking about. Some I recognize from the ER, and they lower their heads in my presence. Others watch me with aggression in their eyes, arms crossed, muscles taut. A rotating guard sits on duty at the end of my hall, beside the linens cabinet, and I have to get too close to him every evening for a clean towel, which makes my heart race. But the rest of them aren't here to transfer patients, and don't appear to be doing anything other than loitering. I don't get it.

My statement was meant to antagonize, to show them I have some power, and it does. The guards react with quick bursts of gruff conversation before scrambling down the hall, presumably to search my room. Moments later, one reappears and says something to Janine from across the room using silent eyes. Her posture stiffens as she's put on high alert.

"Charise, what did you do with the razor?"

Oh. That's what they're worried about. Somebody slipped up and gave me a razor when I asked if I could shave my legs, and now they've realized their mistake. They think I'll use it to attack, although they'll claim to be concerned about self-harm. They weren't concerned about self-harm when I was slamming my head into a steel door.

"I threw it away. It's in my garbage. Do you want me to get it?" I lift a hand casually, to show that it makes no difference to me, because I never had any intentions to use the razor for anything other than its intended purpose, shaving.

"No, that's okay," she says. She looks to the guard who again takes off towards my room, this time pulling his walkie-talkie from his belt and raising it to his mouth. I can't understand him. He's speaking gorilla.

Janine inspects the shallow wound and gives me a Band-Aid. I wander towards the TV area and sit down. Somebody walks past me and sits on the couch, close enough for me to see her sandals and painted toenails.

"Are you okay?" Heather asks. Heather has long dark hair and is always eager to chat. She asks too many questions. It's annoying.

"Fine, thanks."

"How are you feeling? You're looking better," she says.

I'm looking better? She's got a hundred pounds on me, her locks are limp and greasy, and her face is covered in pimples. She's passing judgment on me?

"Thanks," I say tersely. Then I remember something.

"Do you know if they do electroshock therapy here?" I ask. Heather knows a surprising amount about this hospital and its procedures. She often refers to specifics about the schedule, like when doctors do rounds or vitals are taken, and certain rules. Specifics that nobody ever explained to me. I don't know why she's here because she never talks about herself. She doesn't seem sick.

"No, not here," she replies, her voice soft. "But they'll transfer you and do it at another hospital if you request it. Is that something you want?"

She sounds like a waiter taking an order. She sounds like she could make it happen.

"No," I say, firmly. I'm relieved they don't do it here. One of my biggest fears about being locked up is that I'll be forced into shock therapy under the guise of treatment. *One Flew Over the Cuckoo's Nest* and *The Bell Jar* taught me to be afraid.

We sit silently. I'm not ready to return to my room since the guards' invasion. Let their stinky air out first.

"How did you get a razor?" Heather asks. Funny, I didn't see her eavesdropping during the commotion, and I didn't mention that my cut was from shaving.

"From one of the nurses," I say.

Heather nods.

"Which nurse?"

The way she asks this seemingly innocent question, so probing and forceful, puts me on high alert.

"I don't remember," I say. I do, but I'm not throwing that nurse under the bus.

Charlie ambles over and collapses on the other end of the couch. Heather gives me a look, rolls her eyes, and sighs. She doesn't like Charlie. She's told me I should stay away from him because he's a drug addict. I don't know who she is to cast stones. I like talking to Charlie. He's had a hard life but he makes it sound entertaining.

"Time to go, right Charise?" Heather stands and stares into me with bulging bug-eyes.

"I'm good," I say, remaining where I am. Charlie's eyes are closed, so he won't be much of a conversationalist right now, but I'm not eager to follow Heather. Anywhere. She walks away, and after enough time has passed that I don't think she's watching anymore, I stand too. Time to survey the damage.

My room has no specific scent but there's a presence the moment I walk in the door. Like the time when our car was broken into, the glass shattered and radio stolen, and the worst part about it was the feeling that a thief was there, in our space. I feel violated, again, by this hospital. I reorganize everything in my drawers, the closet, and on my window bench, knowing without a doubt that it has all been rifled through with dirty hands. I pack a bag of clothes for Eric to take home and launder, because no way am I wearing anything that's been touched by one of them. I save the bathroom for last, and after cleaning up and purging whatever I can, I walk into it slowly, knowing what I will find. Nothing is out of order. The garbage bin contains soap wrappers, miniature shampoo bottles, and used tissues. The razor is gone.

## 32. The Kindness of Strangers

"You didn't slip in the shower." The cleaning lady whispers. My head snaps up, no longer interested in watching my feet shuffle down the hall. We make eye contact for a brief moment before she looks at her cart and I keep walking to my room.

Her words resonate as I sketch, listen to music, and try to make sense of them. I never said I slipped in the shower, at least I don't think I did. I complained that I wasn't allowed to use the bathroom, but that has nothing to do with the shower. I called them out after that security-officer-peace-man, whoever he is, decided I was a threat after I walked away from him, and forcefully pinned me to my bed. Maybe that has something to do with what this lady, this cleaning lady, this woman who doesn't know me but knows more about me than I would have guessed, felt the need to tell me today in the most subtle way that she could. Because of course they'll blame it on me. My accusation of excessive and unnecessary force will be met with cries of "Bipolar!", "Delusional!" and apparently, "She slipped in the shower!" My accusations will be swept under the rug, unless I have help. And evidence. Like the bruises. And the burning sensation when I urinate, which I mentioned to Janine, who dutifully noted it in my file. Come to think of it, Janine said she would request cranberry juice and I haven't received any. How could that be? Was she humouring me? But Janine is so nice. Did the kitchen mess up the order, like they mess up most of my orders?

So that could be what the cleaning lady is trying to tell me—that people here lie to placate me or get away with wrongdoings, and I'm not just crazy. My thoughts and memories are real and valid too. I don't know exactly what happened on the Friday when I was checked into the ER through to the Monday when I was transferred to the ward, but I know one thing. I didn't slip in the goddamn shower.

I stand from my comfortable window seat and walk to the hall. I feel anger building and need a change of scenery. It's time for a stretch anyway. Too much isolation keeps me too much in my thoughts. My mind gets too busy with things it is best not to dwell on. The trouble is, there's not a lot to do here. There are puzzles, books, colouring books, and a TV, but all of that requires concentration and I'm still not able to focus. There's an exercise bike, but my bruised groin still hurts. I have to ask about going to the gym downstairs, like last year. The workout classes and rock wall felt so good, physically and mentally. I can still hear everyone cheering my name when they noticed I was near the top. It was empowering. That reminds me, I have to ask about group. Last year we did the wall, a drum circle, gardening, and art therapy. This year I've only done walks. Walks are better than nothing, but still. Am I not compliant enough for group therapy? Are they worried I'll tell everyone what happened? Maybe those guards hold the power and they've blacklisted me for everything. Or maybe not, but because of the complaint Eric filed the hospital wants to keep close tabs on me. I'll have to ask, but who? When I mentioned it to Dr. Patel he clammed up. The nurses sometimes look at me sympathetically, but then briskly tell me to go away. I don't get it. Are their jobs in jeopardy if they comfort or support me?

There I go, thinking too much again. Food. I could use food. Food always helps. I reach the kitchen and open the refrigerator door. Egg sandwiches, milk cartons, nothing out of the ordinary. No cranberry juice. I bend down to scan the lower shelves and notice a container of vanilla flavoured soy milk. That sounds interesting. Different. I inspect it to see if it's communal. I can't remember the fridge rules and, like all the rules, they only seem to apply to certain people at certain times. This soy milk is exactly what I want right now. It does not have any obvious markings claiming ownership. I am going to drink this soy milk and no one better stop me.

I find a mug. Patton Oswald and Seth Rogan are rambling about coffee on the TV behind me. It's distracting. A few people mill about or sit in chairs, but most of them look half-asleep. Or catatonic. I open the container, pour out a small amount, and pick it up to take my first sip. It's delicious. It's the first thing I've had off-the-menu of my own choosing up here on the ward. It tastes nourishing and wholesome, better than the green smoothies I buy when Eric takes me to the cafeteria. I want to down the whole thing but Patton and Seth are too annoying. I reach for the cap to close the carton, so I can take my mug back to my room and enjoy it in peace. Only then do I notice the name "Agnes" printed almost illegibly on the cap. I know Agnes. She's from South Africa too. We've shared stories. She's older, so she has more, but she keeps most of them buried. She had a Black mom and a White dad and a very different experience from mine. I look up, across the room, and see Agnes sitting near the window. She's in her own world, so I don't think she's noticed me stealing her milk, and I'm too chicken to interrupt her to give her the bad news. I quickly close the carton, replace it in the fridge, and pick up my mug. I exhale as I walk away, and return to my room to enjoy my drink. But now it's tainted. I tell myself that it's not a big deal, I didn't mean to do it, and throwing it away won't right the wrong and will only waste it, but I still pour it down my bathroom sink. I just feel guilty. Agnes is my friend. One of my only friends these days.

"You have to what?" Eric looks irritated.

"I have to go to a grocery store to buy soy milk." I feel patient but annoyed. Why do I have to repeat myself?

"And, why?"

"I accidentally stole somebody else's."

"You—what?"

I don't understand why this is so difficult. And I'm eager to get out of this parking garage and off hospital grounds.

"Can we go?" Eric's car has been idling during this conversation. I don't like idling. It makes me anxious.

"Oh, yeah." He glances around before pulling forward. "Do you have to go now?"

I'd like to get it over with, but not enough to go now. Grocery shopping is my least favourite chore.

"No, just before I go back." I'm too eager to get home and see the kids. See my mom.

"I don't understand how you accidentally steal something." Eric drives up the ramp and into daylight. He doesn't understand most of what I do.

I lift two grocery bags onto the counter, so the nurse can search them before checking me in. Like so much of what is done "for my safety" while in hospital, this process used to make me feel small. Bringing in personal items is liberating. A way to regain control in a situation where I've lost all control and it's my own fault. Having personal items confiscated strips me of that control. Like so many hospital experiences, it makes me feel like a prisoner, caught trying to smuggle in contraband with impure intentions. Untrustworthy. The nurses never make me feel this way intentionally. They took my phone at the beginning when I couldn't remember the rule or, later, forgot to remove it from my purse. That was understandable. When I brought an alarm clock radio from home, happy that I could now have time and music in my lonely room, it was disallowed. The nurse was sheepish as he vaguely explained that the cord was a safety issue. This was ludicrous from my perspective: either another blanket rule applied to all mental patients without taking into account individual needs, or retaliation for the drama I caused after they let me have a razor or because of my assault complaint. That nurse kindly found batteries and a ward radio for me. He was patient and often tried to help, as most did.

Because I'm used to bag searches now, I no longer take them personally. It helps that I rarely have anything confiscated. Usually I bring clothes, snacks, books, and art supplies. Nothing contraband. Today, this nurse is eyeing my groceries suspiciously. She looks at me, her hand still in one of the bags, her face registering confusion, not discipline, which is a relief.

"Why do you have six boxes of soy milk?"

"Oh, that's for Agnes," I say. My heart starts to thump and I feel like I'm in trouble even though she is very nice and I haven't done anything wrong. At least I don't think I've done anything wrong. I can never be sure. It was wrong to steal, but that's what I'm trying to right. Surely six boxes make up for one small glass?

"I drank hers without realizing it was hers, so I'm replacing it. The prunes are for her too. I didn't take prunes, but she asked me to buy some when I confessed about the milk." I'm babbling and it makes me feel guiltier. The lady doth protest too much.

"I see," she says. She starts to take the boxes out, and the prunes, but she's not angry. "Agnes is on a strict diet. She can't have access to this without supervision."

"Oh." So that's why Agnes told me to give it directly to her. I'm crestfallen. Not only can I not repay my debt, but I've also inadvertently made another mistake they might interpret as defiant or lacking judgment, two of the many characteristics of mania, and Dr. Patel might keep me here longer. I just want to go home, but my privileges and hopefully impending release might now be in jeopardy.

"I'm sorry, I didn't know," I say. "She didn't tell me."

"No, she's clever about it, that Agnes." This kind nurse smiles and it doesn't seem like I'm in trouble, but I can never tell. Many of these nurses seem clever after the fact too. I feel a sudden urge to end this conversation. To remove myself from the line of fire.

"Can I keep the rest?" I didn't bring much food, mostly granola and fruit, but I'd like to keep it if she says it's okay.

She nods and draws the plastic handles together before handing me the bags. Then she quickly looks inside my regular bag, the one containing clothes and magazines, before telling me I'm free to go. I'm reassured by how fast and inattentive she is, believing it to mean that she trusts me and recognizes that I made an innocent mistake about Agnes. Believing that I haven't totally messed up again. She dismisses me kindly, and I walk away slowly, forcing myself to act normal so it doesn't look like I'm fleeing or paranoid or anything. I spend a lot of time these days trying to act normal, both in here and at home, but I'm starting to realize that I don't really know what normal is. I think instead of acting normal I have to simply not react. Stay calm, don't show sadness, anger, joy, or excitement. Don't show weakness. Don't be myself.

"Ah, Charise," the nice radio nurse greets me when I turn the corner at the end of the nurses' station. "It's good to have you back. It's always calmer when you're here."

I nod and say hello, masking my surprise. Did he really say that? What the hell is that supposed to mean? I'm not manic anymore and haven't had any delusions lately. Did he really say that? I sometimes want to ask people to repeat themselves, even write it down, so I have proof. Evidence that I'm not having another psychotic episode. But I don't know this nice man well enough, even if I did have a pen and paper. Or my phone, for a voice recording. There are so many things I could do with my phone right now, so many ways it would comfort me. If only they would grant me even limited access and it didn't cost me something else, like last year when I had to choose between using my laptop off-ward or time spent away from the hospital, with my family. I would never choose technology over my family.

I continue walking, turn the second corner around this U-shaped ward, and notice three security guards standing close to my doorway, as though they're waiting for me. Waiting to entrap me. One of them is the one I nicknamed Irish LEGO guy, the one who attacked me. I am instantly back in that moment in that room feeling the sudden sharp pain between my legs, the heat of his hands on my body as he forced me down.

I don't know how long I stand, frozen, silently staring, and telling myself to breathe before I finally will my feet to move. I cannot let him see that he hurt me. I cannot let him see that he won. I start slowly but pick up my pace until I'm walking at my regular speed. This hall feels longer than it ever has before. I hear a noise behind me and turn to see the nice radio nurse standing where I just stood, a forced smile on his face. If I didn't already know this man, I would freak out, because it feels like he's blocking off my only exit. But we've had many conversations and he helped me with the radio, and I know he has a good heart. I know he's not here to box me in, he's here to watch and intervene if need be. He's here to protect me from the people who are supposed to protect all of us. His presence is more reassuring than he could possibly know.

I'm close now, only a few feet away, and I make a point not to move aside but to keep walking the line, not giving an inch of respect. I smell them as I approach, their awful mix of cologne and testosterone, and I almost brush against the back of the one facing the wall, acting as though nothing is happening even though it's clear that they're here for me. It was clear that they noticed me the second I appeared, and have been pretending to ignore me to bait me into a reaction. I think this burly one whose back I almost touch but have the good sense not to, because I'm sure they'd justify it as another reason to assault me, and I am a mental patient who still sometimes has good sense, is the second guy, the older one, who came into the room and must have pulled Irish off me, but he's too much of a coward to turn and show his face. Irish is the last one I have to walk past, and I feel both anger and fear rise when he turns on an angle, looks at me with cold eyes and a false smile, and waves his left hand down the hallway as though politely granting me passage. As though he owns me. I want to spit on him, yell at him, or say something like, "What a gentleman today," or, "Is that your apology?" or even, "This empty hall sure needs three of you to secure it," but I muster all my strength to stay silent as I glare at him with as much hatred as I can project. I know they're here to provoke me, so they have a reason to justify his assault. I'm not going to give it to them. I can't lose passes or privileges and I can't give him any control.

"Well, that wasn't what I expected," my good nurse says to himself loudly enough for us to hear. No fucking kidding. I make it to my room with four pairs of eyes fixed on the back of my head, walk straight to my window seat, and pick up my sketchpad. I will not collapse. I will not cry. I will not throw or break anything. He would just love that.

# 33. Sad Perseverance

"I know there's nothing hiding, but I'm still scared." Suzie weeps. She rarely weeps.

"Suzie, sweetheart." I rub her back and pull her close. "Shhhh."

It's bedtime and we're in her room. Today I was out on a day pass. It's been over a week since I was admitted to the psych ward. I have to be back in half an hour. Suzie's sitting up in bed with the duvet covering her legs. We've already read her story. It's unlike her to purposely delay the moment where I kiss her goodnight, the moment where I walk away and she's left alone. It is so unlike her that I know this fear is real.

"Sweetie, why do you think there's a monster in your closet?" None of my children have ever been afraid of monsters. Until now.

"I don't know," she says between sobs. I wipe her cheeks and offer a sad smile. Then I inhale deeply and gently blow my breath onto her forehead, something we do together to focus on our breath. She responds with her own deep inhalation and after a moment, blows her breath on me. We repeat this dance a few times, until she is calm and her tears are dry.

"Mommy, do you have to go back to the hospital tonight?" She looks at me with pleading eyes. I don't want to make her cry again, but I can't ignore that this is why she's so upset. I nod and lean in for a hug. She wraps her arms around me and clings on desperately. We stay this way for a while, neither of us wanting our embrace to end. Without moving away from my sweet, sad daughter, I glance at her toys and pictures. Her dollhouse sits beside her bed, the little wooden family arranged as though they're having dinner. Books and larger dolls, gifts from a dear friend as soon as I was hospitalized, lie on the floor. On the wall above her bed hangs her calendar, the one included with the magazine subscription she loves so much. She's decorated most of the page, and seeing her little doodles on Mother's Day makes my heart ache. She's also crossed off all the days up until today, and on each one she's written 'Bad,' or 'Good.' I carefully read her almost-six year-old handwriting. Every day was good until the day I was hospitalized. They've been bad since. Now my heart breaks, and I know I will remember this moment for its sweetness but also for its lesson, for the rest of my life. Any time I'm tempted to defy doctor's orders, or stay up late, or give into the excitement of hypomania, this image of my devastated daughter and her bad days that I caused will remind me to get over myself. To come down. To focus on her and her brothers, and their needs. To do the next best thing. I am hit by a tsunami of guilt, grief, and gratitude all at the same time. I pull back and gently rub Suzie's shoulders, easing her down onto her pillow.

"I don't like it when you go there. I want you here."

"Me too." I kiss her forehead. "The doctor says I have to go back for just a little longer, but I can keep coming home in the day."

"You're not too-fast talking anymore. Can't you just stay?" She stares at me with the saddest eyes I've ever seen.

"I'll be there to pick you up from school tomorrow. I promise."

She doesn't respond.

"Is that okay?"

She nods.

"Want me to sing you a song?"

She nods again. I haven't sung her to sleep in years, but we both need it tonight. I stroke her hair and softly sing her favourite bedtime song, "I See the Moon." I then kiss her on both cheeks, and stand to walk away.

"Love you, Suzie," I say as I step into the hall, turn, and pull the door towards me. Not to close it, never to lock her in, but to make her room dark and quiet while still leaving a crack.

"Love you, Mommy. To the moon and back."

"I'm ready to go."

Eric is on his laptop, trying to catch up on the work I keep making him fall behind on.

"Okay, just let me wrap up," he says.

I put on my sweater and shoes. I packed my bag hours ago so I wouldn't forget anything. This time I'm bringing my own battery-powered radio so I don't have to keep borrowing one. I have a change of clothes for the morning and a few more art supplies, as well as the book I'm currently trying to read. Reading is a problem when I'm manic, or coming down from a manic high, and can't focus, but this time I know it will pass and I'll be able to figure out the plot and characters soon enough. At least I hope so. If the past year has taught me anything it's that I can't give up. I have to persevere. I have to have hope. I have to keep remembering that this too shall pass.

"I'll be in the car," I say as I open the door.

"I'll be right there," he says.

I step outside and am captivated by the mountain ash tree in our backyard. The one Suzie and I agree is hers, because the view from her bedroom window is filled by this one glorious tree. The May evening sun shines on its branches with their buds and leaves, and the light makes it glow. Soon it will be covered in white petals followed by red berries that will fall to the patio, staining the concrete and soles of our shoes. It fills my heart with joy and sadness to bear witness to this beauty, this moment captured by me and no one else. I'm tempted to return to Suzie, for I know she's not yet asleep, and open her curtains so she can admire her brilliant tree. But tonight's been hard already, on both of us, and one more goodnight might be the straw that breaks the camel's back. She needs peace and I need to meet my curfew.

Eric steps out the door and stands behind me.

"Got everything?" He sidesteps around me and gives me a tender smile. I nod and follow him to the car. I close my eyes as he closes my door, and don't open them again until we've pulled away from our home. I hate leaving them like this.

"You okay?" Eric asks.

"Yeah," I nod. "I just can't wait to sleep at home."

"I'm just glad you're not so angry anymore," he says. "And we can spend time together again."

Something about his statement jerks me out of my melancholy.

"When couldn't we spend time together?" I say. He checks his left shoulder before merging onto the highway. What else have I forgotten?

"You know, at the beginning. Sometimes when I visited they told me it'd be better if I left because I was making you too agitated."

This is news to me. They made me agitated by holding me captive, refusing me a toilet, drugging me, and attacking me. Eric's absence made it worse, not better. How could there be so many layers of miscommunication? Was it their plan to drive a wedge between us, because they'd treated me so horribly? By telling Eric I was too angry to receive him, they knew he would walk away dejected and I would have no allies. I suddenly remember the chair that appeared in my room after the assault. The one no one mentioned yet made it seem like they were being nice. Were they really trying to be nice, or just keeping up appearances?

Eric reaches to hold my hand. We're both quiet for the rest of the drive.

"So how was your day?" My nurse digs through my bag, checking for contraband.

"It was great." I mask my emotions. I feel as though I have to stand at attention, as though she's assessing me and whether or not I can handle another day pass tomorrow.

"What did you do?"

All I can think about is that stupid chair and my daughter who is likely crying into her pillow right now or being comforted by my mom. But that's not what this nurse wants to hear.

"I was with my family," I say. Then I remember something I can offer to appear normal. "I was packing."

Her eyebrows arch up, giving her the appearance of someone who is on guard. My heart beats slightly faster to warn me that her reaction means I need to be on guard too.

"Why were you packing?"

"We're selling our house," I say. I think this is the calmest, most sane-sounding reply.

"You are?" Her eyes bulge. I need to tread carefully because although I know I am telling the truth, they have accused me of delusions before when I was telling the truth.

I nod. I wish I hadn't mentioned it. Thank goodness Eric is still here to corroborate my story.

"Have you bought another house?"

"No." I hope she stops questioning me. If I tell her we're moving back to Toronto in less than a month after making the decision mere weeks ago, she will surely declare me insane. And in trying to persuade me to tell her the truth, I will lose privileges like my passes, my belongings, and my room. I can't go back into the high-surveillance room again. It is torture.

"I'm really tired. Can I go?"

She looks over my shoulder, at Eric, for verification. He nods and gives her one of his charming smiles. Her eyebrows drop and her serious expression returns.

"Okay, here you go." She returns my bag. "Dr. Patel will be here in the morning between nine and ten. He can assess if you're ready for discharge."

My eyes open wide and I allow myself a small smile.

"Can you be here?" She asks Eric. "It would be best to have a family meeting." Eric reassures us both by saying that he'll be here, of course, and then turns to me to say goodnight.

"I'll see you in the morning, okay?" He looks into me with love and concern. I nod. We hug and he kisses the top of my head. My eyes fill with tears but I blink them back.

"Don't believe them if they tell you not to visit. If they say I'm too angry." I speak softly into his chest, with my head tilted up, so the nurse won't hear. He pulls back and kisses my forehead, but doesn't reply. Then he turns and walks away. I don't know if he heard.

"It's great you had a good day," the nurse says. "Tomorrow should be just as good."

I nod and breathe deeply.

"I'll bring you your meds shortly."

I nod again.

"Thanks," I say.

I walk away, feeling like the woman in that IKEA commercial yelling at her husband to start the car because she thinks she's about to be stopped, because she got away with such a good deal. I got away with telling the truth and not being reprimanded for it. If only I could tell Eric to start the car. If only we could drive off, get away from this place.

## 34. Stifling All Urges

"So many people," I say as my nurse Sarah, Dr. Patel, and two other staff members file into the meeting room where Eric and I sit. I say hello to the ones I recognize, but am stumped by a pleasant looking woman who could be a doctor, a nurse, a peace officer, or all of the above.

"I'm sorry but I don't know you," I say as I shake her hand.

"This is Dr. Lee, Charise, you've met before." Dr. Patel says. He sounds surprisingly stern.

"Oh." I try to recall when we've met. She smiles patiently. "Perhaps in Dr. Patel's office?" There are often students at my appointments, in fact the other unknown person here was introduced to me as his articling student. No that's not right. Interning something or other. Some sort of underling whom Dr. Patel is training. A padawan.

"You've met many times." Dr. Patel directs Dr. Lee to a chair and sits in the empty one beside her, next to me. He looks at me with a blank face. "Let's get started."

I force my nervous lips to smile, at least partly, and wait for him to speak. I think we're here to discuss that I'm ready to leave the hospital, ready to go home to my loving family, but now I'm not sure. We've never had so many people at our meetings, so it feels more like a firing squad than a celebration.

"We are here to decide if you are ready to be discharged." Dr. Patel remains stern. He is usually in a better mood. I nod again, too nervous to let my voice betray me.

"Do you feel that you are ready?"

I start to speak, proclaiming my affirmations, until he looks from me to Eric. I end my sentence and softly take a breath. Eric backs me up, basically repeating what I've said, and it's what my psychiatrist wants to hear. His solemn gaze starts to soften. I take this as a cue that it is okay for me to talk, and repeat the last thing Eric said. Dr. Patel looks at me. He seems annoyed that I've spoken. Apparently I am no longer allowed to advocate for myself. I remain silent and listen to them discuss my fate. Again. I interrupt when somebody says something I disagree with, and receive a cold glance from one or both of them when I do. Sarah, the student, and Dr. Lee all remain silent. Eventually Dr. Patel turns to me.

"I am concerned, Charise, and I'm being completely serious here."

I nod and bite my tongue.

"I am not sure that you are ready to be discharged. You're still showing signs of pressured speech. I am not convinced that you will take your medicine."

I feel like I'm fighting for my life here, but he only sees pressured speech.

"I know you have excellent support and I can trust Eric. But I'm still not sure."

I lied to him once. And now he thinks I'm completely unreliable.

"I will take it," I say softly. "Whatever you prescribe, I will take."

The conversation turns into a discussion about my medication. Too many pills and too many details for me to pay attention. They'll let me know once they've made their decision.

"You take the synthroid between meals, correct?" Dr. Patel asks.

Which one is synthroid? Oh, right. Thyroid. Nobody cared about my hypothyroidism when I struggled to get pregnant, but now it has to be dutifully monitored. They say it's caused by the lithium, and ignore me when I disagree because it's always been wonky.

"I take it at bedtime," I say. "With the others." Dr. Patel's head jerks back.

"Together? No, no, no, Charise. That cannot be. It should be early in the morning or between meals. And never with dairy." He shakes his disappointed head.

"I don't understand," I say slowly, thinking out loud. "I've been doing that the whole year. No one mentioned dairy. Even here, they give it to me in the morning, but sometimes at breakfast, while I'm drinking milk." I look to Sarah for confirmation, her word to back up mine and prove I'm not the feeble invalid they think I am, because she did this very thing, watched me swallow my synthroid with a sip of milk, an hour ago. Sarah avoids my eyes, pretending to be occupied with the hem of her sweater. Guess I'm taking one for the team. Again.

Nobody looks at me. Nobody acknowledges what I've just said. Instead, they discuss how my pills should be prepared so I will take the correct dosage at the correct time. I'm no longer reliable enough to even count pills, apparently, let alone comprehend their timing. Even if I buy myself a pillbox and even if I write it all down. I am no longer at all reliable.

"Okay, I'll do the blister pack." I repeat whatever Dr. Patel says. At this point I will say and do anything to get out of here.

The conversation continues, to satisfy everyone present that I am stable enough to be released. Eric makes a joke about me playing with fire because of my Chinese zodiac animal, a dragon. It's the sort of joke I would be reprimanded for, but he's not crazy, so everybody laughs. I stay quiet to prove I am in control of my speech. My silence pleases them. I am dismissed. And discharged.

Back in my room to pack before they change their minds. I only have a few belongings this time, so it won't take long. Last year I had enough clothes and supplies to last months, because everything was so uncertain. This year I asked Eric to switch out my clothes daily and only bring in the bare minimum: books, writing implements, an old iPod, and art supplies.

There is a loud knock. I turn to see someone whose name I never caught standing in my doorway, holding a vase of colourful flowers. It strikes me as odd that I don't know her name. She's in the room beside me, a room I walk past many times, but unlike every other patient, hers has no name card. I want to call her Debra. She looks like a Debra.

"I'm leaving today so I wondered if I could give these to you?" Debra says. She stays where she is, obeying the rule that patients cannot enter other patients' rooms. I like this rule. It makes me feel safe. While walking over to meet Debra on the threshold, I recall an image from a few nights ago when she was in my room along with a nurse, the good nurse who was my hallway protector. He was putting batteries in the ward stereo I'd borrowed, and Debra asked if that was the source of the beautiful music she'd heard late at night. I apologized for disturbing her, but she insisted that I hadn't. She said she enjoyed it. I wonder how she came to be in my room, when that is the only rule they strictly enforce. It strikes me as odd.

Debra has not been here long. I noticed her bed in the hallway beside our rooms, draped with an expensive-looking quilt, a day or two before she arrived. I wondered who the VIP was and why she warranted pre-made coziness before checking in. Half of the time my "bed" in the ER didn't even have sheets. We've talked many times; conversations with Debra are calming. We once watched a movie together, *Braveheart*, and gossiped about Mel Gibson, like friends having a ladies night in. Yet I know nothing about Debra or why she's here. There is nothing obviously crazy about her. I don't know why she was given a special bed. Or was allowed to chat in my room. Or is here giving me her flowers, because apparently she's being discharged at the exact same minute as I am. I don't know why, but I have a theory. I think she's a spy. I think the hospital planted spies to keep tabs on me. I thought this last year too, but in hindsight I could have been paranoid and delusional. This time, however, some of the patients truly don't seem like patients at all. And this time, we've filed an "unnecessary roughness" and possible sexual assault complaint against the hospital. And this time, they're taking extra precautions to make sure certain rules are followed, like Dr. Patel won't talk to me alone in a closed-door room even though our past year of appointments have often been behind closed doors, alone. Yet other rules are dismissed, like another patient being allowed in my room. I'm sure they have explanations for the peculiarities I've noticed—they are as good at explanations as I am at noticing peculiarities. Especially when they can blame any oddities on my overactive imagination or psychotic delusions.

I take Debra's flowers without a second thought, because it is such a kind gesture. We both wish each other well. It is only after she walks away that I realize I should not have accepted them, because I too am leaving. Why would I want Debra's flowers in my home? I wouldn't.

Eric has finished packing during this exchange. I stand frozen, staring at the bouquet in my hands.

"Ready?" he asks.

I look over.

"What should I do with these?" I hold the vase at arms-length, as though the flowers are already decaying. As though they might burn me.

"I don't know. What do you want to do with them?" Flowers have never been Eric's strong suit.

"I guess give them to the nurses?" That's what we did with my bouquet last year. I thought it would brighten everybody's day. They seemed appreciative.

"Are you ready?" Sarah asks as she walks into my room. I want to confront her about not backing me up in the meeting, but it's not worth it. Just another betrayal for me to accept. At this point I can't remember how many times they've betrayed me to save themselves.

"We're trying to figure out what to do with the flowers," Eric says. He raises his eyebrows at Sarah, as though he's asking her to take over before he loses his patience. The request seems too much for her.

"We're doing what now?" Sarah's face contorts into a question mark. I start to explain, but before I finish she takes the vase from my hands and walks to the nurses' desk down the hall. I follow her, curious about their fate.

"Let's put those here for now."

I'm confused. Nobody sits in this spot, so why would we put them here? I start to protest, but Sarah insists that she'll find a good home for them. Eric has my bag. Sarah gently but firmly steers me towards the lockers. It feels like she wants to get rid of me, either because I am a nuisance or for my own good. If I don't take the chance to leave now, who knows when they'll grant me another one? And then I notice something.

"Why does that sign always say today is Wednesday?" It hasn't changed since I arrived, ten days ago.

"What?" Sarah turns. "Oh, right. We should really change that."

An oversight? That's all it is? We rely on that sign. Something so important in our screwed up world that doesn't merit any importance in theirs. I want to voice my dismay, insist that if they're going to put up a sign that's supposed to help us, then at least have the decency to not add to our confusion, but now is not the time. I'm getting out. We arrive at the lockers and find the good nurse, my protector, waiting for me. He greets me and turns to open my locker. I expect it to be empty, because lockers are for safekeeping confiscated items or cigarettes, but it is not. It contains one single item: my family photograph encased in its cracked frame. I haven't seen it since LEGO guy broke it, and the sight makes my heart hurt. I tell my protector I don't want it, it's broken and tainted. He tries to persuade me to take it, but my mind is made up. We have plenty of pictures at home, and I have hundreds more in my supposedly defective mind. I will never look at this one without seeing pain. It's ruined.

Sarah buzzes the maglock to let us out. We walk out the first security doors, wait to be buzzed through the second security doors, and quickly make our way through the hospital to the parking garage. Driving away, I feel like we've escaped and we're getting away with it. I try to put the uneasiness out of my mind and focus on the fact that I am free, that I get to be with my family without being on a clock. My mind keeps turning back to those flowers. I wonder what Sarah did with them, if anything. I can't shake the feeling that she threw them away.

## 35. Selling Our House

I set down a glass of water on the table next to Richard Jones. He is busy typing but nods his thanks. I sit on the chair between him and Eric, and Eric pulls our chairs together. He reaches for my hand and holds it in my lap. I guess he wants Richard to know we're a team. Us against the world, or something. I did not expect to be meeting with our real estate agent so soon after checking out of the psych ward. Eric must have mentioned it to me, but my mind still has so many holes. I'm too tired for this.

"Okay," Richard says. He turns his laptop towards us and starts his presentation. It looks professional and informative, but we've bought and sold two houses, so it feels like a waste of time. He runs through the package like it matters. I guess it does, but not really, because we are moving no matter what, and we are getting rid of this house no matter what, so most of what we discuss today is essentially moot. I'm not sure why Eric is paying so much attention.

"This is what I mentioned to you on the phone, Charise," Richard says, pointing at the screen as he elaborates on something I don't remember. I smile and nod and chime in every so often, so he feels appreciated. I do appreciate him, and the work he's doing for us, so I'll waste my time pretending to listen if it makes him feel appreciated and do a better job. This is part of the game we all play.

I glance at Eric, whose face is stern. My husband often wears a stern face. It's difficult to tell if it's because he's concentrating or annoyed. Richard notices too, so he tilts the laptop towards Eric and begins to address him more, to give him his attention. I can see why Richard is such a successful real estate agent: he reads people as well as I do.

I start to squirm. Richard is showing Eric comparable after comparable and we just don't need everything. Especially because most of the comparables aren't even that: comparable. Most of the houses are older and unrenovated, or renovated but tiny, or renovated but huge, or backing onto the lake. Nothing like our house has sold in the last six months.

"I see," Eric says. He pulls his hand away, leaving mine lonely in my lap. "So, this is relevant to us, Reesie, because to calculate our asking price we can compare it with the list price and selling price of these houses."

Duh. We only learned that twice already when selling our previous homes. Since when does my husband speak tenderly to me in front of a stranger during a business meeting? And since when does he explain something he thinks I don't understand in front of someone? Eric's been wanting to show Richard Jones up ever since he met him. He was surprised that I called Richard Jones weeks ago, before going manic, about selling our house, even though we discussed it and agreed that I should action it. He didn't think I would do it. He was further surprised that we had an efficient and entertaining conversation. The alpha-male behaviour Eric is displaying right now would be amusing—even flattering—if it didn't feel so condescending.

"I got it," I say. I give him a look that likely goes over his head. "I'm pretty sure Richard did that already to come up with this number."

"Yes, I did." Richard nods. "But, Charise, if you'll look at this for a moment." He turns the laptop and starts to ramble about why I should care about all the work he's done, because obviously I don't, because obviously it makes no difference to the bottom line. We're moving in two weeks. We need to sell this house as soon as possible, for whatever we can get for it. The list price Richard suggested is reasonable in this market. Eric doesn't like it because it's lower than he wants. And he always likes to work a better deal anyway. And he's not a big fan of Richard right now. This cockfight is wasting our time.

"I've got to get the laundry." I rise abruptly, stomp to the basement stairs, which are only a few feet away so stomping is not particularly effective, stomp down the stairs, also not effective since they are carpeted, and walk into the laundry room. I open the washing machine lid and peer inside, but then remember that this was an excuse. There is no laundry. I had to get away from the men so they could finish trying to outdo each other without needing to vie for my attention. I open the dryer door and slam it for effect. Then I slam the lid on the washing machine in case the first slam wasn't dramatic enough. Then I rehash our conversation to delay going back upstairs, and it hits me that maybe neither of those men in my kitchen are acting kind and attentive because I'm attractive. Maybe they're explaining things I already know and treating me like a princess because I just got out of the hospital and they think they need to wear kid gloves. They think I'm an idiot. Just because my mind is tired doesn't mean it's broken. I slam both the dryer door and washer lid again, like a child having a tantrum, because I'm so frustrated. Frustrated at Eric for treating me like I'm stupid, frustrated at Richard for pandering to Eric as part of his job, frustrated at both of them for wasting my time and making me so angry that I had to leave and hide downstairs. If I hadn't just been treated for mania and released from hospital I would be concerned that my anger and confidence about my knowledge and sexuality, are signs of hypomania. But I'm medicated. And sleeping. I'm not manic. Sometimes feelings are just what they are, even for bipolar people.

I head back upstairs, feeling slightly better. Hopefully they are done. I hear laughter from both men before I reach the kitchen. I left them alone for ten minutes and they became best friends. What a cliché. Eric spots me in the doorway. He doesn't look concerned for my wellbeing even though the look on my face can't be good and he must have heard the laundry room rage. I guess he's concerned enough to include me in our real estate conversation, but not enough to inquire about my feelings when I'm obviously upset. Or he is simply strutting, because it was just a cockfight and had nothing to do with my bipolar stupidity.

"Oh, good, you're back. We still have a few more things to talk about." He extends an arm towards me.

"I'll see you guys soon." Mom's voice calls out from the mudroom. I hadn't realized she was there. I notice the clock on the stove. It's almost three o'clock. Almost time to get the kids from school. Perfect.

"I'll be right there, Mom," I say loudly. Then I turn to Eric. "We have to get Jack and Suzie."

He gives me a look, like he knows something's up because my mom is perfectly capable of doing school pick-up on her own. This is the second spring she's rescued us. But Eric doesn't say anything. Maybe his look means nothing.

"Do we need Charise here, Richard?" Eric asks. I've already walked to the mudroom and don't hear Richard answer, but I also don't care. These men seem incapable of getting things done with me around, let them figure it out while I'm gone. Besides, they'll waste time analyzing every little point until I get back and can sign whatever needs to be signed, with whatever stupid details they've agreed on, which won't matter at the end of the day. I look at my mom, roll my eyes, and shake my head. She smiles and puts an arm around my shoulders even though she doesn't understand my body language. She's just happy to have me home from the hospital. She's just happy that life is almost back to normal again, at least for now.

"Okay, bye," I say as we walk out the door and I close it behind us. Mom adjusts Piper's leash.

"Ugh, perfect timing, Mom. I had to get out of there," I say. A walk and fresh air and Calgary's blue sky is exactly what I need right now. It's exactly the antidote for everything. I can't believe we'll be leaving it so soon.

# 36. Goodbye Dr. Patel

I hear my name and turn to see Dr. Patel standing at the waiting room doorway, staring straight at me. He once told me that my "intense" eye contact was a symptom of mania, which made me laugh. I am an intense person. Almost everything I do is intense, at least everything that matters. And if intense eye contact is a mark of insanity then Dr. Patel needs to check himself. He has the most intense eye contact of anyone I know.

We nod our hellos, and I tap Eric's arm as I stand up. If Dr. Patel is pleased to see me, then he is delighted to see Eric. His smile broadens, revealing perfect white teeth, and his eyes light up. This makes me bristle, and I have to silently remind myself to stay calm. It's difficult for me to feel anything other than irritated when these two men are together and I'm the third wheel. But as I've been told, irritability is a symptom of my illness. I have also been told that my illness makes me overly sensitive. So my reactions are sometimes attributed to my illness before being dismissed, at best, or preventing my release from hospital, at worst. I have to fake it till I make it, at least when my husband and psychiatrist are in the same room. Dr. Patel greets Eric like a long-lost friend and then turns to me, his patient. The reason for our gathering.

"Good morning, Charise. This way, please."

He holds the door for us and gestures towards his office down the hall. We walk into the room and sit down. Dr. Patel's office is surprisingly small. It is barely large enough to fit his wrap-around desk, built-in bookshelf, ergonomic chair, and two visitor chairs squeezed between the desk and the door. Books line his bookshelf, but he has few personal items on display. I notice that the bodybuilding caricature is still pinned to the bulletin board, along with some thank you cards. The room has no window, only an overhead fluorescent light.

It feels stifling. I can't imagine sitting here to work all day. But I guess people can adapt to anything. It could be worse.

"When can I stop the olanzapine?" I say. Dr. Patel adjusts his shirt sleeves after settling into his chair. I'm not supposed to be talkative so today my plan is to stick to the point. It'll be hard. I love to talk when people pay attention.

"Why the rush?" he asks once he's comfortable.

I sigh inwardly. We've been over this. He knows my answer. He knows how I feel about olanzapine: it makes me groggy and fat. I notice that Eric is watching, ready to step in if he feels I'm steering the conversation the wrong way. I am both annoyed that I need his surveillance and relieved to have his support.

"I'm gaining weight. It took me so long to lose it last time."

"I don't see it." He gestures towards my midsection. "It's not noticeable. Besides, you could afford extra weight."

"Yes." Eric nods. "That's what I say too."

I resist the incredible urge to roll my eyes. The two of them get like this when they're in agreement. Like a father and an older brother deciding the fate of a young girl. Not that I've experienced that firsthand. My father and brother never ganged up to control me.

"Yes, that's what I'm told," I say. "But I know it's there. I feel heavy and clumsy. Besides, I don't like these drugs. They make me sluggish and uncreative. Sometimes I twitch. Sometimes I feel nauseous. And the acne on my neck has been awful." I am self-conscious as I say this, and relieved that my long hair conceals most of the ugly, red pimples.

"That's not from olanzapine. You haven't been on olanzapine that long." His response is matter-of-fact. He's right, but it's irritating. I just want to regain control of something that is happening to my body. Something that is happening to my life.

"I read that lithium causes acne," I say. I have to tread carefully because this was one of the reasons why I decided to decrease my lithium before I went manic. But I don't want to remind these men of my betrayal. Neither of them have forgiven me. Neither of them trust me.

"It can make an existing condition worse. It does not cause the acne." Dr. Patel replies quickly and dismissively, as though it doesn't matter that the drugs make it worse. As though it is a separate problem that I must simply accept.

We stare at each other as though it's a draw at high noon. Finally, he gives.

"Charise, I'm reluctant to stop the olanzapine with the stress of moving to Toronto, especially since you don't have a psychiatric team in place. It cannot simply be stopped anyway. You will need to be weaned off when the time is right."

He thinks he's got me, but I was prepared for this.

"On that note, we brought referral forms to ask you to fill in." I pull a folder from the bag at my feet and pass it to Dr. Patel's outstretched hand. I explain that each form is for a Toronto hospital that has been recommended to me because of its psychiatric services. He looks over his glasses at the two of us, and back at the papers, before nodding and picking up a pen. Eric gives me a look that I read as him telling me to stop talking. So I do. We sit there, the three of us, in a silence that feels awkward to me. I watch as Dr. Patel patiently completes each box, occasionally checking my file for accuracy. Hopefully this will not be in vain. I don't know if an Alberta psychiatrist can make a referral to an Ontario hospital, but his efforts give me hope.

"We should have filled in the basics," Eric says. Dr. Patel doesn't hesitate, merely continues with his neat printing. I guess Eric's feeling the quiet pressure in this room too. It feels like we're asking too much, taking too much of his precious time. Dr. Patel has never done anything to make us feel like our time is less valuable than his. He has never once rushed me. But we all know how many patients need him. How many patients are waiting for him, watching that clock above the nurses' desk until he arrives on the ward and starts making assessments, doling out passes and privileges. Inpatients and their families are waiting to learn if they can leave because Dr. Patel is diligently taking his time to help me. I sure hope it's worth it. I sure hope it helps me find a new psychiatrist.

"How long have you been planning this move?" Dr. Patel asks after returning the completed forms an eternity later. I hesitate, hoping Eric will answer so I can demonstrate that I have control over my speech. I also want Eric to explain so Dr. Patel knows this move is not a whimsical manic impulse, lacking judgment and insight, nor a desire to spend excessively or take unnecessary risks. I want Dr. Patel to know this idea was not mine and the decision was not mine alone.

"It just came up," Eric says. "My boss asked me at the beginning of May."

Dr. Patel's eyebrows shoot up, forming a valley of wrinkles on his normally smooth forehead.

"Just one month ago? That is sudden." He looks at me. His eyes are thoughtful and imploring. He looks concerned, as he often does, but in a way that is more considerate. It's not his typical urgent, self-assured concern, like when I'm manic. It is more worried and uncertain, because he won't be able to help me. He looks like a parent sending a child off into the world knowing that the world will be cruel and there's nothing he can do.

I tune out. I hear snippets about packing, the upcoming road trip, the importance of managing my stress and keeping me medicated, and our future living arrangements. We could have delayed the move and taken time to gently ease our way back, but we like to dive headfirst. Eric does not want to buy a house sight unseen, so the faster we get to Toronto the faster we can find our next home. Until then we will live in a hotel or with my in-laws. I'm not looking forward to it. I need my own space to feel settled.

"How do the children feel?" Dr. Patel asks.

"They're fine," I say. Eric glances at me before turning back to Dr. Patel.

"It's a lot for your family. Especially with the timing." He gestures towards me with his right hand, the one still holding his pen. This makes me feel small, like being bipolar is a cross that my family has to bear and it's my fault. Which it is.

"I want you to be very careful to manage your sleep, Charise. It is critical for you to stay on your medications."

Yes, yes, I've heard it before. I've been lectured so many times about the same thing that the words have become meaningless. I simply nod, because my vocal reassurances are a waste of time here.

"Eric, you will need to go with Charise to her appointments so you can make sure her new psychiatrist truly understands." Dr. Patel stares at Eric with his intense eyes. "She is very persuasive. *Very persuasive.* Do not let her persuade her new psychiatrist into weaning her lithium for at least one year."

This statement, and the fact that he's speaking as though I'm not in the room, frustrates me. I am very persuasive because I am logical and my arguments make sense. They are honest and well-intentioned, not deceptive and selfish like he makes it sound. I'm not a used car salesman convincing families to spend all their savings on a lemon. I breathe deeply so I won't react, because I'm not allowed to be argumentative or grandiose for fear of repercussions: more lectures, more prescriptions, possibly more hospitalization delaying our move. I work to control my facial expression.

"Does that mean I need the higher dose for a year?" I ask. A month ago, Dr. Patel increased my regular 900mg of lithium carbonate to 1200mg, to compensate for my reduction to 600mg. Lithium can be toxic in high doses. While hospitalized, my blood was regularly tested to monitor my lithium levels, but I won't have this luxury until I find a new Ontario doctor. Which could take months. I ask my question because I need the answer, but also because I need to focus on something other than my apparently sneaky persuasion skills. I wonder if hyper-persuasivity is one of the many symptoms of mania. It's another "symptom" that is fine for "normal" people, but since I have the bipolar label people get their backs up. Especially my husband and psychiatrist.

Eric gives me a sidelong glance. I can't read his expression perfectly but I think it is one of pleasant surprise. I think he's somewhat impressed that I'm with it enough to ask this question. To be honest, so am I. This last month has been hard, and my current drug cocktail makes me foggy, just like last year.

"No, you will have to get regular blood tests once you have a doctor, my dear. You will be able to reduce to your regular 900mg under supervision." Dr. Patel says 'my dear,' when he's pleased or upset with me, like when I phoned him to say I hadn't been taking my medication and might be manic. He replied, "You did this to yourself, my dear," with frustration in his voice. He is smiling now, so he must have liked my question too. It's a sign of my ability to perform daily tasks. My ability to function.

"But, Charise," he says, "you must report if you have manic symptoms. You must not hide symptoms. And after weaning, you must stay on 900mg for at least one year and only reduce at that point if you have a psychiatrist's approval and supervision."

Another year of lithium would have sounded like a jail sentence a few months ago. Now, after my failed experiment, I don't care. I don't know how it works or how I was okay without it for forty years, but it doesn't matter. At least not now. I need to be stable for my family more than I need to eliminate a drug that could help and hopefully isn't causing long-term damage. Olanzapine is another story though. I haven't needed it for this past year, since weaning off after my first hospitalization with Dr. Patel's approval, and am not willing to take an unnecessary drug indefinitely, especially one that has such ugly side effects. Even my family doctor told me to get off olanzapine as soon as possible.

"Okay, Dr. Patel. I'll do that. But what about olanzapine? Can I wean off that over the next few months like last year?"

He purses his lips and shakes his head, but his eyes are smiling and he's suppressing a grin. I am lucky to have this kind, good-hearted, hard-working man take care of me, even if he does prefer my husband. I will miss him and his support when we leave Alberta. Despite my initial misgivings when we first met, I have grown to trust him. If only I'd met him before going crazy things might have been different. For both of us.

## 37. Moving Day

It's been a month since I was hospitalized and only two weeks since I was discharged. Today we leave our Calgary community of three years to return to Toronto. The 6ix. Hogtown. The Big Smoke. *Home*. I feel nervous.

"What are you doing?" Eric asks. I didn't hear him sneak up on me. He probably wasn't sneaking, just quietly observing me moving around the dining room.

"Just looking at everything the movers will pack," I say. They're coming in a few days to box up our lives and bring them to an Ontario storage facility. One of Eric's office assistants will supervise. "Wondering if we need it all." We've accumulated a lot over the years. It's always cathartic to purge.

"Too late for that. We leave in an hour."

I stare, transfixed, at my diploma. Bachelor of Engineering, Honours Mechanical, McGill University. The red border. The school crest. The ugly brass frame I purchased knowing it was a mistake, to match Eric's from his graduation one year before. When I graduated we were planning our future, and we liked the idea of matching diplomas on our new apartment wall. Over the years mine rejected its frame and the paper began to warp. Not that it matters. This self-important document has collected dust in the basement of whatever house we've lived in since we first bought a house. I don't know if it's worth keeping, since my engineering career seems to have abruptly ended. I feel like it's mocking me. Without this piece of paper I would never have met my husband, but do I really need to treasure it for that reason alone?

"Did you sleep okay?" Eric asks.

I snap my head back into the present moment. He has a way of inquiring about my sleep that feels like it's more doubt than concern. Like he's not asking for my wellbeing, he wants to know if he needs to brace for another storm. It's the same when he asks if I took my meds. It was the same last year after I was first released from hospital, so I don't think it's just because of my deceit. I don't know what it is, but it's unnerving. I don't think I'm reading too much into his tone, but he would likely disagree.

"Yes. Why?"

"Just wondering. You're up early."

I look for my phone, but it isn't here. My heart skips a beat at the realization that I haven't been vigilant enough about time and might have lost more, after all these weeks trying to put it back together.

"What time is it?" I ask, reluctant to admit that I don't know. I cannot show weakness.

"Six-thirty."

I exhale slowly. That's a good time. No need to worry.

"We leave today?" I ask. He nods.

"And today's June the eighth?"

He nods again. He's never sure how to react when I ask him these questions—the ones that reveal the black holes in my mind. My need for reassurance troubles him, and then he needs reassurance. I don't know if he's getting it from anyone. He doesn't like asking for help. This is why I avoid asking him questions or discussing my research and theories. I know it'll unsettle him. And he doesn't want to hear it. He doesn't want to be unsettled. Fair enough.

"Perfect." I look at the notepad and pen in my hands. "I made this for the new owners."

I give it to Eric, hoping for his approval. Canada Post began using community mailboxes and stopped delivering to our door shortly after we moved in. There are a number of bulk mailboxes nearby, and I don't know how the new owners will find their mailbox, unless we share its location. Presumably they could contact Canada Post but also presumably the answer would require some patience and effort. This is the thought I woke up with this morning, the one that coaxed me out of my comfortable bed. I've written down its location, and added a sketch of two community mailboxes side by side with an arrow pointing to our/their box, showing its close proximity to a nearby school. It's more of a doodle than a sketch, but it still pleased me to draw and I'm happy with how it turned out. I wouldn't call it creative but at least it's not entirely uninspired. Plus, it will be useful.

Eric takes the notepad from me and studies it before returning my gaze.

"Good idea," he says. "This is good." From the look on his face he is pleasantly surprised that I thought of this detail that no one else, not he, not our real estate agent, thought of. And I acted on it. That I'm once again becoming independent, capable, practical.

"I'll make breakfast. The kids will be up soon." I smile at him because I feel proud of my little doodle. Proud that I've done something to help make the transition easier for the people who will take over our lovely home. Proud of what this means for me in my recovery.

Eric smiles back. Then he stops me for a hug as I walk past him on my way to the kitchen. It's a good one: tight, long, and I feel him inhale as he buries his face into my neck.

"You smell so good," he whispers. I squeeze him close before I walk away.

I watch my children play on their playground one last time. Jack dangles upside down from the bar connecting the rings, flipping and repositioning every few minutes. Suzie swings. She would swing all day if she could. Alex sits on a swing, dragging his feet through the dirt below. He enjoyed this playground when we first bought it, after Eric and I struggled to assemble the tunnel slide and I had to lie in the dirt with ants crawling through my hair for him to force pieces together at the right angle. It's the most frustrating thing I've ever built, after a career assembling finicky and intricate lab automation. It was worth it.

"Okay, guys, look at me!" I lift my phone, poised to take their picture. Jack and Suzie smile big, goofy grins. Alex looks up, but his face remains neutral. I guess him being twelve years old isn't the reason why he doesn't want to swing. He wasn't happy when we told him about the move. Jack and Suzie are thrilled to live close to grandparents and cousins again, but this isn't enough to console Alex. He has real friends here.

"Let's get some in front of the house," I say, shepherding them through the side gate to the front porch. We take a few shots and I manage to coax a smile out of Alex, and then Eric announces that it's time to go.

"We've got to get on the road if we want to make it to Regina with enough time for a hotel swim."

I force everyone to make one last bathroom trip before we pile into the car. They grumble, but they do it. We've packed our essentials to survive the next few months, before we have access to the rest of our belongings again, so suitcases and backpacks fill every vacant spot in our Armada, which we bought recently to replace the truck.

We drive past the front of the house to say goodbye one last time. Alex is silent, staring forlornly out the window while Jack and Suzie eagerly wave and chirp their farewells. The Calgary sky offsets the black shingles and neighbouring pine trees splendidly, as it always does. I will miss that sunny blue sky. And the mountains. And the moon. The huge, luminescent Calgary moon. Toronto's nature, despite its impressive fall colours and spectacular plethora of ravines leading to the lake, just doesn't compare. At least the winters aren't as hard, and our family is there. And I might be able to work again. And I already have friends. I will miss my friends here. It took me a while to form friendships and now that I have, I am saddened to go. I'm glad that none of the children have mentioned leaving the dog behind, with a family who loves her more than we ever did. I will think of Piper fondly although I can't say I'll miss her. She is wonderful, but she added too much stress to my already full plate.

We head down the street and into the uncertain future. We don't have a house. I don't have a psychiatrist. Or a family doctor. Or any idea what school my children will attend in less than three months when summer vacation ends. Or any idea what we will do to entertain ourselves for the foreseeable future while living out of our suitcases. My assault complaint against the hospital, or, rather, Eric's complaint on my behalf, is unresolved. They are supposedly investigating. I don't know what will happen to the investigation once we leave the province. Dr. Patel gave me medication to last a few months, but I'm not sure what I'll do if I haven't found a doctor when I run out. I'm not going to a new ER.

The kids have fallen silent in the back seat. Eric merges onto the highway and reaches across my lap to squeeze and hold my hand. My heart is heavy. I'm eager to leave Calgary, this city where I miscarried so many years ago while on vacation, and where I never thought I would return to visit let alone live. I lost my first baby here and also my mind, and I'm still sad. It's been a short, difficult three years, but it's also been a terrific adventure. What will life in Toronto bring for us all? I feel nervous about this bittersweet departure, but more than that what I feel is relief, because I'll never be back at that hospital and I'll never have to see those security guards again. We're finally fleeing, like I wanted to the first time I was hospitalized. I'm finally escaping their grasp.

Three days of driving and we're still only halfway there. Canada goes on forever. The children are excited and sad, I'm overwhelmed and exhausted, and Eric is constantly trying to put a happy spin on everything for our sake. He must be worn out.

I dutifully take my nighttime medication: lithium (mood stabilizer), olanzapine (anti-psychotic), and clonazepam (epilepsy medication prescribed to help me sleep). I now take the synthroid (for my hypothyroidism) in the morning. The boys are in bed reading, Suzie is lying on an air mattress under the desk at her request, and Eric sits up in bed beside me, on his phone. For once I think I'll fall asleep before all of them. I should have asked my doctor about sleeping pills years ago. This hotel room is so big, well designed, and clean. The air feels fresh and the pillows are perfect. I look at my cozy family before settling down into my covers. I'm too tired to read, and too ready for sleep. I've finally learned to choose something to think about before I close my eyes, so I don't feel anxious the moment darkness hits, and I don't start thinking about something that sends me into a tailspin. Tonight I choose Suzie's birthday dinner. Watching her eat her Worms 'n' Dirt. Watching her open presents. I'm ready. I close my eyes and start to relive the moments. It doesn't take long before my mind drifts to that altered reality, that in-between state of consciousness where I'm aware enough to know that I'm about to fall asleep and have to let it happen without getting excited by the realization and waking back up. I have to give in to my subconscious and let go of control. I focus on my breath to let it take hold.

"Reese," Eric whispers as he gently shakes my hip. The room feels dark. Quiet. It must be late. My eyes struggle to open. I know Eric would never wake me unless it was critical. The kids must be okay or his voice would be urgent.

I roll onto my back, and force my eyes open. The room is dark. A golden light cascades through the cracks between the windows and the heavy curtains, and there is a white glow from Eric's laptop propped open on the desk. It is bright enough for me to see Suzie asleep below the desk, her dark curls splayed in every direction across her pillow, and both arms stretched up above her head. She sleeps just like me. I hope that's not a sign of bad things to come.

"Reesie." Eric looks awake and extremely serious. It's like someone has died.

"What time is it?" I stall. I'm not ready for bad news. I pull the duvet under my chin and blink a few times. I hope Eric knows I'm trying.

"It's late," he says. "Listen, I've been talking with Janet about the house. I'm thinking of putting an offer in."

Oh. That's all it is. Not bad news. I would feel more relief if I was more awake.

"Okay."

"Do you want to buy this house?" He leans closer, eyes boring into mine.

"Which house?" Janet, our good friend and Toronto real estate agent, has been diligently searching on our behalf for weeks. Eric and Janet have discussed some houses in great detail, taking FaceTime tours as she walked him through each one. I think I was there for some of these showings but I could be wrong. I lost interest early on in the conversations, after Eric said he wasn't comfortable making such a significant purchase online. I didn't want to get invested in a home that would be sold by the time we returned to Toronto. Plus, my mind is cluttered and the specifics began to overwhelm me. I remember images of kitchens and backyards, but nothing I thought he had any desire to purchase.

Eric tells me the address and when that isn't enough to trigger my memory, begins to describe it. This doesn't ring any bells but I play along. I feel like I should know which house he's talking about and I'm not sure if my mental illness is a valid excuse for why I don't. I don't want to add more stress to this move by frustrating him because he thinks I'm not interested enough or committed enough or something enough. If he's game, I'm game.

"I think I know the one," I say as I search my sleepy brain for an image similar to what he's described. "Is it that house where they didn't show the picture of the ensuite but the main bathroom was kind of beige and had a skylight?"

He looks at me and cocks his head to one side, and I can't tell whether I'm right, and he's impressed, or I'm wrong, and he's impatient.

"Yeah, I think so." He slowly starts to nod. "I think that's right."

As with many of our experiences, we remember different aspects about the same thing. We focus on different details because they make an impression on our unique needs and desires. I don't remember the furnace room he's described, but I do remember how bright the bathroom was. I wondered if it was because the lights were on but it seemed brighter than the other rooms, which also had lights on, so I read the real estate blurb. It listed skylights as a feature.

"I think there was more than one skylight. Maybe in the kitchen?"

He nods again.

"You're right. The kitchen does have a skylight."

I try, but I can't remember the kitchen. Which is a pity since that's where I'll spend most of my time. I don't love cooking, but it's a big part of my job.

"And it had the big washer and dryer? And the laundry room had those built-in cabinets?" I'm pleased by how much I now remember about this house. It's nice to be reminded that my mind can surprise me in a good way. "What schools would the kids go to?"

We talk about schools. From Eric's eager description, they sound as good as or better than the schools our children have previously attended.

"Okay," I say.

"Okay as in yes?" His eyebrows arch.

"Sure. Yes. If you're okay with putting in an offer then we should put in an offer."

"Really? You think so?"

"It sounds great. Good neighbourhood. Good schools. Close to your work. It's the right size. Expensive but manageable. Doesn't need renovations. We'll move in and get settled soon. Let's do it."

I still haven't shifted from my position under the covers. He leans down and kisses me on the forehead, tenderly squeezing my shoulder. Then he sits back up and starts to talk about the list price and what he's planning to offer. I don't care. We've already agreed on what we can afford and although this house is more than we were hoping to spend, it's comparable with similar Toronto houses and fits within our budget. Eric is much more financially savvy than I am, and much more particular about settling on what he considers to be the right price, so I'm satisfied that he will be more than thorough enough for both of us.

I wait for him to finish talking and when he asks for my opinion, I basically repeat and agree with what he just said. It sounds fine. He looks nervously excited. I feel relieved and tired. I'm ready to go back to sleep. One month ago I was in the hospital and since then we've sold our Calgary house, packed up to move into a hotel, and now it looks like we're buying our next new home sight unseen while on a cross-Canada road trip. Should I be hesitant? Is it crazy of us to operate on such whims? Will my next psychiatrist tell me that this purchase demonstrated overspending and poor judgment, two symptoms of mania? I don't think that's what this is, since Eric is the one driving the decision, and he's not crazy. I wonder momentarily if I should express these concerns to Eric before he texts Janet and tells her to make the offer, but the truth is I don't feel concerned. This feels fine. This feels like something we would have done before I was diagnosed as bipolar, like how we quickly and efficiently made the life-changing decision to move our family to Calgary when presented with the opportunity. This is not as big as that. It's just a house. It'll work out.

## 38. Sort of an Apology

"My name is Monica. I'm the manager for Adult Addiction Services."

I've been waiting for this call. I raise a finger to my lips to silence my children. They smile and nod, happy to lounge on the hotel beds and have unlimited screen time for the duration of my conversation. I walk into our adjoining room, with its king-size bed and assortment of wet bathing suits hanging in the bathroom, and close the connecting door. They'll open it if they need me. We've lived here for two weeks and these rooms are a mess, but I suppose that was inevitable. At least there's a hotel pool, and with no camps or friends or activities, we are grateful for that. Only another month until our new house closes. I can't wait.

When Eric filed our complaint against the hospital we were initially put in contact with Tara, the Patient Relations Coordinator, who seemed sympathetic and supportive but couldn't do much. She passed us to Justine, who works for Alberta Health Services in Edmonton, for the security guard part of the problem. Justine's title is Provincial Manager, Process Improvement and Operational Support, Protective Services. She seems nice enough but it doesn't feel like she's trying to resolve our case. I've had to repeat facts more than once and she, or they, still make mistakes. Maybe it's intentional, a way to cover their tracks. I don't know. I was recently informed that I would be getting a phone call from Monica, the most senior person responsible for "the incident" on the nursing side. I wasn't told that Monica was the manager for Addiction Services. I don't know how that makes her the manager for the ER Psych ward, or whatever its proper name is. But I've been waiting for this call. I'm eager to speak to someone who can provide some answers. I guess that means the manager of Adult Addiction Services, even though I've never had an addiction in my life. I guess they don't care about the stigma, so

I have to pretend there's none. Somebody has got to start thinking about the terminology they throw around with mental health patients, as though it makes no difference. As though it means nothing. As though we mean nothing. Maybe that's their point.

"Can you tell me in your words what happened while you were here?"

"Sure." My voice cracks, betraying my otherwise calm demeanour. I tell her how I was ignored for so long that I had to use the drain as a toilet. "After I fell asleep, a nurse came in and said he needed to check my vitals. I was later told his name is Darren. He acted surprised to discover, in his words, 'a turd.' He cleaned it up as if it was no big deal."

I'm skeptical that the nurse's name is Darren. I inquired about him when I saw him on the ward a week later, and the staff member I asked responded in a way that suggested a lie. I don't think they are obligated to tell me anybody's name, and it might be preferential to give a fake name instead of allowing themselves to be vulnerable. I can understand if they can't divulge personal information, because nurses have rights too. But if lies slip off their tongues so easily, how am I expected to believe anything they say? Perhaps they are lying to me about names and perhaps they are lying to each other about what happened. Perhaps between the nurses and protection services there have been so many lies that nobody knows the truth any more.

"Yes, that incident was charted by a female nurse but she wrote that a male nurse cleaned it up," Monica says. "Well, I am sorry about that. That should not have happened. You were quite sick and it was our job to help you." The word 'sick' gets my back up, and it doesn't help that she doesn't sound sorry. She sounds matter-of-fact. Insincere. Placating.

"I appreciate your apology however it would be more meaningful if it came from somebody who was actually at fault."

There is a pause. I don't hold my breath.

"That's not going to happen," she says.

"Right," I say. I decide to rock the boat. "I've been wondering, is it common to lock patients in their rooms for so long?"

She sighs.

"I wouldn't say that it's necessarily standard to keep a patient in her room unless she's deemed a safety threat to others or to herself."

A safety threat to herself. I was repeatedly ramming the steel door with my head, and that wasn't deemed enough of a safety threat to myself for them to open the door. Even she knows her answer is weak, not that she would admit it. Her job is more precious than one patient.

"Can you tell me what drugs I was given? In addition to my regular ones, I mean. I lost so much time between the Friday when I was admitted to the ER and the Monday when I was transferred to the ward." What I'm really asking is if I was given so many drugs that I can blame them, and not my bipolar mood disorder, for my blackouts and hallucinations.

"I don't have your file in front of me but I did flip through it and I think the only extra drug you were given was Ativan."

This surprises me. I know Ativan is anti-anxiety but can it cause hallucinations? It also surprises me that she doesn't have my file on hand. Another alarm bell goes off. How can she be certain of any details without having my paperwork available?

"Do you know what the doses were?" I need answers.

"I can find out, but it was likely given as necessary. It's a PRN."

I don't know what that is.

"What's a PRN?"

"*Pro re nata.* It means the drug is given as needed at the discretion of whomever is in charge. Doctors prescribe Ativan for agitation or aggression. You also received a few extra doses of olanzapine from what I can recall."

A few? I don't react well to a single dose of olanzapine. It makes my brain foggy and my muscles twitch. It makes me angry. She does not know the answer when I ask if there is a maximum dosage of Ativan or olanzapine, or if there are any contraindications with lithium, synthroid, or clonazepam, replying that she will have to check or I could ask Dr. Patel. So it seems they locked me in my room and when this, and their drugs, made me agitated, they medicated me until I was numb and forgetful. They may as well have given me electroshock treatment.

"You can request to see your chart if you'd like to know what medication was administered." Monica's tone has changed. It's like she's doing me a favour and wants appreciation. I jump at the offer, because it gives me a glimmer of hope. I gratefully thank her as I write down who to contact for this request.

"There's a fee for your health records," she says. "I think it's twenty-five dollars."

Twenty-five dollars is nothing for answers. Proof of what happened to me.

"About the possible sexual assault. Do you still believe that happened?" she asks.

Loaded question.

"I don't remember a lot of that weekend. I don't remember any meals, for example, and I don't remember my family visiting me on Mother's Day, when apparently I was furious." This hurts me to admit. I think it must be my mind's protective mechanism not allowing me to remember. Or it might have been their wicked drug cocktail. "But I do know that a security guard pushed me down from behind and kneed me in the groin, twice, and it hurt for days." It still hurt after I started to remember everything that had happened, both real and delusional, and my mind started making sense again. After the nurses and security guards were no longer administering whatever drugs they decided were appropriate. Whatever dosages they could get away with to blur the lines with a mental patient.

"Well, as you know, I wasn't there so I can only look at the charts and rely on what my nurses tell me. But based on their reports it just doesn't seem like there was a time when it was possible."

Her words provide no comfort. She is relying on her staff's testimony. Their word against mine. Again. What are the cameras even there for, if not surveillance and evidence?

"Have you heard from the Manager for Protection Services yet?" Monica asks.

I say that I haven't, and I've been told that I won't. Tara, the Patient Relations Coordinator informed me that I won't hear from the hospital's Protection Services Manager because the assault complaint has been transferred to Corporate Affairs Investigations. They will mail us the results. I hope they take it seriously and use surveillance footage instead of relying on guards' stories, like Monica with her nurses. Otherwise it's my word against all of theirs.

"Well, as I said, it just doesn't seem possible."

This is the vaguest answer that she could give. I would love to be relieved by proof that I was not assaulted, but claiming that it's unlikely because there wasn't an opportunity and her employees say it didn't happen is just total bullshit. All she's done is leave more room for doubt.

"Well, that would be great if it's true." I linger on each word and the sentence comes out intentionally frosty. This conversation has created more loose ends than it's tied up. I don't know what else to say. Apparently neither does she, because there is a long pause before she speaks.

"Dr. Patel would like to know how you are doing and if you've connected with psychiatric care in Ontario." Much like her offer of my health records, this sounds like an attempt at a peace offering. It sounds like she wants to move on and leave things on a good note.

"That's nice," I say. And it is. Dr. Patel expressing concern for me now, after everything that's happened between us and when I'm no longer under his care, means a lot. "I'm doing well. My mental state is stable. I found a family doctor surprisingly quickly and I've been referred to a psychiatrist. Please thank Dr. Patel for asking." I don't mention that the referral appointment will be months away, and I've been told to head straight to the ER if I need immediate care, because that's the fastest way to see a psychiatrist in Ontario. I don't think that's the kind of update Dr. Patel wants to hear.

I know she wants to wrap this up but I'm not letting her off the hook yet. It feels like this is my only chance.

"Can you tell me about a shower? I have a memory of someone waking me up and washing my legs. I was a mess and too drugged to clean myself." Somebody wanted to help me. It might have been Eric. Or somebody wanted to hide evidence.

"I can certainly check your file. There is no shower on that ward, so it would definitely be written down if you went off-ward for a shower. Somebody from protection services would have had to be there, but they wouldn't have helped you because they're not allowed. They can only stand guard."

This is not comforting. Guards aren't allowed to touch naked patients, but they can watch? And also, I was in the ER from Friday through Monday and they don't have a shower, so they just expect patients to adapt to our filth? What I really want to know is why I was woken from a deep sleep supposedly to check my vitals and, later, to clean my legs, when what I needed was the cocktail of medication Dr. Patel figured out last year (which they did not give me in the ER), proper care, and sleep. Last year I was taken for an MRI in the middle of the night, which was urgent to rule out other issues, and understandable timing because that machine gets busy. But to wash? And vitals? Why would those be deemed essential enough to wake me when I was finally asleep? I decide to ask.

"Why would I have been woken up to check vitals and clean up? Doesn't the staff know to let a sleeping manic patient sleep?"

"Yes. As I said, I have no knowledge of a shower. Vitals are required."

Her voice is cold and distant. If I were her, I would feel uncomfortable and repeatedly apologize to a patient who was mistreated. I would feel remorse. She is not uncomfortable. She does not feel remorse.

"Is it typical to give a patient in the high observation room a recliner after confiscating everything and refusing to open her door?" I'd almost forgotten to ask her about that cushy chair that appeared in the corner of my shithole room after the assault. It barely fit. The chair was either an attempt to apologize, or something they could use to fool my family into thinking they were taking good care of me. Something they could use to discredit my claims of abuse. It worked on Eric—he was impressed that they were trying to make me comfortable. The guards were full of misinformation, like telling Eric to go home because I was too angry, when I needed his support because of their mistreatment. Since I was furious, Eric took their words and actions at face value. He was fooled. It made me more upset.

"I wouldn't say that's standard procedure, no," Monica says. Her curt reply indicates that my time is up.

"I would appreciate any facts about the shower. There is so much about that weekend that I'm still piecing together."

"I know, and I would just like to reiterate how sorry I am that you were kept in your room when you needed the bathroom. That is unacceptable. I will be reviewing that incident to see what rules we need to change and I will have a conversation with the nursing staff about letting a person out when they need the bathroom."

This sounds genuine, despite her lack of emotion throughout our conversation, but it's also absurd. What kind of nurse requires such instruction? What kind of person requires such instruction? Still, it's a step toward what I want, toward what I've been asking for since Eric filed our complaint. Because I've decided that I don't want anyone else to go through what I went through. I want the mental health care system to change to treat patients with dignity. I want the tired, complicit staff who don't see us as human beings anymore to be made more aware and less ignorant. I want those things on the big picture. But what I personally want—right now—is an apology from the people who hurt me directly. Recognition of their wrongdoing. Genuine attempts to understand the impact of their actions, and a pledge to do better. I would feel guilty if I were them, even if I convinced myself that I was just doing my job and it was the right call. I wonder if they feel guilty. I wonder if they ever think about how hurtful and hateful their actions were. I wonder if they know how frightening it is to feel your own mind going crazy, and the difference that being kind and gentle can make. I wonder if anyone really knows. If not, maybe I should speak up.

# PART THREE: *Hope*

*August 2018*

## 39. Facing Demons

Eric pushes the front door open, steps aside, and waves me through, so I can be the first to enter our new home. I step onto marble tiles and slide out of my Birkenstocks. The floor feels surprisingly warm on my bare feet.

"It's so bright!" My voice echoes. I turn and almost crash into Eric, who has silently crept up on me. We laugh.

"It really is bright," he says. He wraps an arm around my shoulders and we survey our new kingdom. The house faces west and it's early in the day so sunshine pours in through the back windows, flooding the open concept main floor. It gives me confidence that our midnight, online, sight unseen decision was a good one.

We explore each room together, parting to focus on whatever appeals to us and then reuniting to head through a doorway to the next room. The children are with Eric's parents today and overnight, so that when the movers arrive we can focus without being distracted. This gives us an unfettered freedom: no snacks, screens, Star Wars, or Strawberry Shortcake issues to navigate. We roam the house from top to bottom, returning to the main floor once we're done. There is a fresh, excited feeling in the air—*we own this*! In the kitchen, I stare up through the skylight while Eric tests the water pressure at the sink. The finishings are not our style. The pelmets, wallpaper, gold-beige palette—all of it is too European, too elegant for us. We like simple and modern. Grey. This décor feels fussy. It was renovated a decade ago, and it shows. It doesn't matter. None of it matters. This house will serve us well.

"I'm so glad you bought it," I say. "This house is great."

"Me too. It really is," Eric smiles, pulls me towards him, and we share a long embrace.

"I can't believe we pulled it off," I say. "It feels like we just got back, but we already have a house, a family doctor, and my psychiatrist lined up. Everything is working out. I haven't felt this kind of flow since being manic."

Eric goes pale and I realize the implications of what I just said. I need to calm down.

"Not everything is perfect, Reese. You didn't get your job back, remember? And the movers screwed up our van."

I nod. My former boss was certain I could have my job back, but it didn't work out. And the moving company wrecked our van door during delivery, so now it's in the shop. Both disappointing. But both good reality checks.

"You're right," I say. "Not everything is coming up roses."

We smile.

"When are the movers supposed to arrive?" I thought they would be here by now and am eager to start. I've been rearranging furniture in my mind for weeks.

Eric checks his phone. They're half an hour late.

"I'll call," he says. I sit at the marble table to wait. The built-in booth is comfortable, but this corner is dark. The window has an exterior awning to cover the deck, which is accessible through the door beside the window. Unfortunately the awning throws a lot of shade, and the result is a moody space. This will be where my children spend countless hours eating, doing homework, and creating artwork, so I'm disappointed by the lack of natural light. I remember something my favourite boss once said when we were trying to work out a few software kinks: nothing is ever perfect. It was a statement more about life than robots. We can take down the awning.

The phone call is not going well. Eric is flustered and saying things like "That wasn't what we agreed." I rest my head back. There's nothing I can do but tell myself that everything will be fine. Eric will work things out. He's good at getting what he wants.

He starts talking about rescheduling and it's obvious the plan has fallen through. The move is not happening today. He finishes his call, angry but holding it together well enough to appear calm. He's good at that too.

"They messed up the date," he says. He begins to rant about our incompetent moving company. I wait for him to finish, knowing from experience that this is the best course of action. Once it's out of his system he will easily move on.

"What's the new plan?" I say once he's done.

"They're coming tomorrow."

Okay. Disappointing, but okay. There's nothing we can do and it's just one day. We have our essentials and Eric wisely brought his guitar, so I can look forward to an extra-long performance. It's not the end of the world. Nothing is ever perfect.

"Do you want to sleep at my parents' house?" Eric asks. We've spent most of the day relaxing and reconnecting, some much-needed quality alone time. Almost like a date.

"No," I say. "We've always stayed in our house on the first night." I think back to Oakville, when the builders were staining the stairs on the day we took possession, so we had to sleep on the main floor. Our Bloor West house was easy: our movers set up the beds and I'd conveniently packed the sheets so that after a long day we would sleep well. We flew to Calgary for that house closing a month before the actual move, so we slept on an air mattress even though the alternative was a fancy hotel on Eric's company's dime. We unknowingly started a tradition, one I'm determined to continue.

"Okay," Eric says. "We'll have to get an air mattress from my parents. I can go alone if you want."

"No, I'll come. Do you want to go now?" I miss the kids when we're apart and besides, what am I going to do here with no furniture, internet, or food?

"It can wait. I should do some work."

"Okay." I smile. With nothing specific to do, I wander aimlessly until I end up in our new bedroom. Our new sanctuary. I glance around the hollow space. I figure out our furniture arrangement here, and can picture myself propped up against the headboard to read before bed. Our dresser will sit against the wall beside where I stand, facing the bed. The baby pictures will sit atop it, along with the vase from my grandmother and perhaps a plant. Something green. Along the wall we'll hang children's artwork and our wedding picture, the one where amongst the chaos of the day, Eric silently watched me from across the patio. The one that makes me feel like he only has eyes for me. I see all of it in my mind, but the only thing I see in real life is my Eureka backpack resting against our suitcase on the floor. I pick it up and start to open it, but then I remember that it contains my notebooks from both highly creative manic episodes. I've avoided looking at them until now, because they show my true madness, and I'm reluctant to sift through them here, in this room that will always need good vibes for me to sleep. Maybe it's silly, but I want to keep this room fresh. No bad memories.

Yet it feels like it's time to explore my past, the inner me. I've focused on the hospital, research, science, treatment, and the future. Now I need to look within. Understand my perspective during my manic episodes. Face responsibility. There must be a reason why I kept these items close to me, with me, instead of packing them in a box with everything else. There must be a reason I have this free time in our new home. I need to unpack myself before I can unpack my family into our new life.

Holding the backpack at my side, I carry it through the house. Eric notices me walk past.

"I'll be ready to go in an hour, okay?" he asks.

"Sure," I say. I pull on the back door, which sticks before it opens. If I were overthinking I would see that as ominous foreshadowing, but I'm not, or at least not right now, so I remind myself that it's just an old door.

"Do you want my hotspot for your phone?" Eric says. My hand reaches for the storm door handle.

"Maybe later," I say. I prefer not being connected sometimes. No temptation to scroll social media, no ability to send or receive emails. I look at him, surrounded by his work at the kitchen table. We share a smile. "Thanks."

The deck has no furniture and no comfortable seating area. I head toward the edge, where a step allows me to sit with my feet on the ground. I gently place the backpack down, slide the zipper open, and carefully pull out my stack of memories.

The first notebook is small, its footprint less than the dimensions of a sheet of paper and barely half an inch thick. It is mint green and the cover is embossed with cursive gold script that reads "This is the beginning of anything you want." It was a gift from a friend shortly before my first mania. Remembering her makes me smile, but I flip it open and the first page wipes the smile right off my face. I see a vibrant mix of crayons and pen, doodles and symbols with a few words spread out for clarity. I remember doing this at the beginning of my mania, thinking I was recording genius ideas and explanations for the meaning of life, religion, and world peace. I think if I could decipher the code that seemed logical at the time, it might make sense. But I don't know the code when I'm not manic, and I can't decipher anything. The journal looks exactly like stereotypical ramblings of an insane person. Utter madness. It shocks me to see how crazy I was. To know that without doing ALL OF THE THINGS (medication and an extremely structured fitness and eating regimen and daily routine that prioritizes sleep), I could be that way again in a matter of weeks.

I wonder if I should stop myself before turning the page because it might upset me, but I feel more curious than upset. I flip through the pages, which contain similar sketches, equations, and explanations, and before I know it that first book is done. There are two more, but I know they won't be as difficult, because they won't be the first. The first book, depicting the first mania, was always going to be the hardest. And it's done. I looked at it and I'm fine. I pick up the second book.

It's a spiral-bound workbook that belonged to Jack in grade two. Prior to my second mania, I began using the blank pages as my journal. I flip through from the beginning, chuckling when I see some of his artwork, and feeling the familiar heartwarming glow of mother's pride. This is a nice buffer between my last journal and what's to come, and I take a moment to savour it. But then Jack's work ends and my work begins. Unlike my previous journal, this one is written almost entirely in pencil and is mostly words. There are a few doodles and shortcuts to explain my theories, but these pages do make sense. To me. I've written down various theories about parenting, diet, exercise, and even mental illness. I remember creating this. I told Eric it was a blueprint for a series of books I would write. I'm surprised by how logical everything is considering it was written one week prior to my second hospitalization, just three months ago.

I pick up the third and final book. It's a proper artist's sketchbook, a gift to Alex when he was too young to appreciate it. Each page is thick and feels satisfying. Luxurious. This one I still use, but I've never gone back to look at the beginning. It has art from my first hospitalization up until today. Some of it is raw, like the colouring page of a dragon that I decided to make more fierce back in the first psych ward, because that's how I felt. Some of it is stunning, like my onion flower or the page Jack described as zentangling after I finished doodling it. I don't know what that is but apparently my children learned it at school. I was just doing what came naturally. I flip through each page, feeling both pride and shame. It's impossible to deny that my best, most creative, artwork is from each time right before my mania turned bad. I recognize this with a sigh, and a heavy heart. But then I sit up straight and tell myself it's okay. I miss creating my best art but I don't love being manic enough to do it. At the end of the day, I'm only creating it for myself so it doesn't really matter how good it is. It does matter how sane I am. It does matter how present I am for my family. It does matter that I continue with this plan to medicate and sleep, stay healthy, draw and write and sing, and recover.

I feel sunshine on my neck and look up at the trees in our new backyard. This is a peaceful backyard. It's shady, I don't know if we'll be able to grow tomatoes like we used to before Calgary, but it's peaceful. Lots of trees. The one in front of me is split in three, which reminds me of my children. Any trio makes me think of my children. There's a lone, tall oak a few feet away, and another oak beside me, growing through a hole in the deck specifically built to accommodate it. It's split into two but still the strongest one here.

The door behind me creaks open and Eric steps out onto the landing.

"It's gorgeous out here!"

"Yup," I say. I stack my journals together and slide them into my backpack. I feel relieved to have that over with. I don't want to get rid of them, they're a part of me that I want to protect, but I won't be afraid to look at them anymore.

"Ready to go see the kids?" Eric says. I pick up my backpack, stand, and turn towards him.

"Let's go."

# 40. Needing Support

My fingers stop flipping through the mail after landing on a letter-sized envelope addressed to me. It does not have a return address, but is stamped with the word 'Confidential.' I turn it over and see the words "Health Information Management" on the back, suggesting that this slender envelope can only be one thing. My health records. I thought they would require a manila envelope. I feel a twinge of disappointment. I open it and pull out a handful of papers. There are eight sheets in total, including the cover letter. I sit cross-legged on the floor, relieved that the kids are busy unpacking toys and will not interrupt me, and begin to read. The first page, after the cover letter summary, is an Emergency-Urgent Care form dated May 11th, 2018. It must have been when I was admitted. It contains mostly illegible handwriting although I can make out words like "agitated," "delusional", "rambling speech," and "clanging thoughts." The second page is an outpatient consultation dated May 12th, 2018. It is a doctor's summary that doesn't tell me anything I don't already know. Some of the descriptions, like "grossly disheveled," make me cringe, but then I read the line, "She maintains very intense eye contact," and I laugh. Has this physician ever met Dr. Patel? The next page is a Multidisciplinary Progress Record dated May 13th, 2018. It is covered in messy handwriting and medical shorthand, so I cannot decipher much. I was admitted on May 11th and transferred to the psych ward on May 14th, so it seems this page might be a summary of my treatment or behaviour on the Sunday of that weekend, although it's unclear because it is so difficult to read. Where is the summary of the Friday and Saturday, when they refused to let me go to the bathroom and physically assaulted me? Where is the summary of the drugs they fed me for those days? Don't the nurses make file notes too? The next page is an outpatient consultation from Dr. Patel on May $14^{th}$, shortly after he assessed me in what I call the ER, the Emergency Room, because it was the temporary stay until a bed opened up on the ward. On this form it's called ED-Emerg. I have heard it referred to as the Acute Mental Health Unit, Acute Inpatient Unit, and now also Emergency-Urgent Care. It would be helpful if hospitals and staff could simplify unnecessary confusion—they seem to have no idea how hard our brains are trying to work. This page is another summary that is mostly familiar but one line jumps out, "She still remains pressured and elated despite the fact that she has received a lot of p.r.n. medications." A lot. A fucking lot. Nice to know there's some small proof. The last three pages are lab results and a discharge summary by Dr. Patel's student. Again, I laugh when I read, "It was a pleasure being involved in Charise's care. We wish them the best going forward." Such a nice sentiment. It's like I was at a spa.

I rifle through the pages again, reading each one in more detail to see if there's anything I missed. I read words like "euthymic," and "labile," which don't help me much. My health records apparently have no record of anything that happened to me on May $11^{th}$, aside from admission, or May $12^{th}$. So, either they weren't documenting the drugs and treatment over those two days, or they intentionally removed that paperwork from my file. What's even worse is that this false hope cost me twenty-five dollars. I feel duped. Something that was supposed to comfort me and resolve my questions has only made me more suspicious. I remember Monica saying "The incident was charted by a female." There's nothing here about that, or anything from those two days. Monica used the words chart, records, and file interchangeably, just like they use different labels for the ER and switch between the terms security guard, peace officer, and protective services officer, as though purposely trying to confuse and distract me. There is nothing here about the feces, like Monica said there would be, or the Ativan or olanzapine or anything else they gave me whenever they felt like it. Did Monica intentionally mislead me? Or did someone tamper with the evidence?

I pause at the bottom of the basement stairs to decide if this is a good idea, and to work up my courage. I want to turn around and climb back up the carpeted steps, keep walking out the back door in the corner of the kitchen, and avoid this conversation altogether. When Eric got home from work, I told him about my health records, but he was dismissive. It usually means something when he's dismissive. In this case, I think it means he wants me to drop it. Move on. I think his dismissiveness reveals not only disinterest, but also disbelief. Things between us have been tense all night.

I walk into the rec room where Eric watches TV. He looks up.

"Do you want to resolve this?"

He shrug nods. I take it as permission to sit on the couch. Not beside him, I leave the middle seat empty. We both need space.

"I feel like you don't believe me," I say. He's watching that comedian he likes, the one who jokes about food. It's good background noise.

"I know that's what you think but I can't control what you feel."

I take a breath.

"Do you believe me?"

"It's not about whether I believe you or not. I don't not believe you."

I don't know how he thinks that's an acceptable answer.

"That's not the same as believing me," I say.

He sighs.

"Some of what you say happened is so impossible that I don't know what to believe."

I nod. Watch the guy's routine. He is so family friendly. The kids love his bacon jokes.

"I believe something happened with that security guard," he continues. "But then you tell stories about patients who were secretly staff planted there to observe you, and the nurse who was watching porn on his computer. It just starts to sound surreal."

"I don't think they were planted there just to observe me," I say.

He stares at me like I'm crazy. Like I'm literally crazy right now, which I'm not.

"Is it so hard to believe that they want extra eyes on patients to assess their mental capacity based on what they do rather than what they say?" I challenge.

"You think they have the money and the time to have dedicated staff playing dress-up just to watch what's going on in the psych ward?"

"Maybe. How do you know they don't? Maybe it's volunteers. Or students."

He shakes his head.

"I think it's unlikely," he says.

*"He must be mentally ill,"* booms from the television, the comedian's shrieking voice cutting into my thoughts. Wait. What? I glance at the screen. This comedian, who doesn't make fun of anybody except himself, is making fun of mentally ill people. Making fun of me. And the audience is laughing like it's the most hysterical thing ever. Ha, ha, ha. I reach for the remote and switch the television off.

"Unlikely doesn't mean impossible," I say.

He turns to look at me, staring deeply into my eyes.

"When I was in the psych ER, people kept mentioning the name Andy. I can't remember who or why, but they kept saying things like 'Who's Andy?' or 'Tell us about Andy.' Like they knew I had a relative named Andy and were fishing for me to say something specific. I don't know what. When I arrived on the psych ward, I met a patient named Andie, and that alone didn't trigger anything, but then I heard her story, which was long and complicated and had serious coincidences with mine, and then I noticed the name written on the paper beside her door kept changing. It was always Andie, but every day the spelling was different. One day it was A-N-D-I-E and then A-N-D-Y and then A-N-D-I-Y, and so on. Finally, near the end of my hospitalization, so long after they could accuse me of being delusional, it was spelled A-I-N-D-I-E-Y. Bizarre. So, I asked her how her name is spelled because it keeps changing on her sign. Deer in headlights. She recovered and asked me how it was spelled on her door. I spelled it for her. She replied, 'That's how it's spelled,' and that was that. I went to my room for something, and when I came out she had the piece of paper sitting on the table beside her and was reading a book." *Watership Down.* She recommended it to me many times.

He's been staring at me intently through my story.

"Does that not strike you as odd?" I ask.

"Yeah, it's odd. But it's a mental ward," he says.

I sigh again. Of course that's the easy excuse. Maybe Aindiey was a patient. Maybe, like that comedian said, we're all mentally ill, so ha, ha, ha. Maybe the nurses kept misspelling her name, or she had her own reason to change the sign, and it had nothing to do with me. But there were so many inconsistencies in the psych ward. Too many to ignore them all.

"What about the security guard who pretended to be a patient?"

"You don't know that. Maybe he was there because someone called security."

"He was wearing the gown they force us to wear when we've done something wrong and they want to shame us by taking away our clothes. He was pushing a janitor's mop, which we're not allowed to do. He was behind the nurse's station, where we're not allowed to go. He was having a private conversation with his nurse when I interrupted, and the nurse allowed me to stay, which is also not allowed."

"Okay, so, yes, all of that is weird. But I still don't think everything you said is believable." He doesn't add, "Because you're mentally ill," because he knows enough to realize that it's cruel. Ha, ha, ha.

"The hospital knew we had lodged a serious complaint and you don't think they'd want extra eyes on me? They asked you what I wanted, like I was going to sue them for millions. Nobody, not even Dr. Patel, would be alone in the same room as me. He's been alone in the same room with me for the past year!"

"Maybe, I don't know. I just don't know."

We stare at each other searchingly. This impasse feels deadlocked.

"Tell me again what happened," he says.

I tell him again, elaborating on anything I might have previously left out. I don't tell him about unrelated things, like when moss began to grow out of the wall or when I saw holograms of him and the kids reflected from the security cameras. I've never told anyone about those hallucinations because I know they weren't real. And that makes them embarrassing. Makes me more crazy. But somehow it is comforting that I can recognize what was and what was not my trickster mind. It reassures me that what happened with the security guard isn't all in my head. And also, there was physical evidence from his attack.

"I was bruised for days. Even after I was transferred to the psych ward and being properly taken care of and not so angry or manic. I thought I had a UTI because it was so uncomfortable."

"I know. I remember you talking about it."

"So, do you believe me?"

"Yes. I believe something with the security guard happened."

He has no idea how relieved I am to hear those words, vague as they are. To have at least one person believe me, sort of.

"But, do you think you might have done something to provoke him?"

I stare at him blankly. The momentary relief I felt is replaced with disbelief.

"Of course! I was manic! They locked me in that room and I was furious! I could have been hurling insults and calling him names the whole time. For hours! But I was never physically aggressive to him or anyone other than myself. And when he attacked me it was after I'd returned to my room, walking away from him to a confined place where they'd been holding me captive. How is that cause for his reaction? Because I was being defiant by not obediently following him at that exact second? He couldn't have given me one minute to explain myself given my fragile mental condition? If they know I'm manic and keep telling me I lack good judgment, how can they physically attack me for lacking good judgment?"

"No, you're right, it doesn't justify his actions."

"I get that I'd been poking the bear and he exploded. So, my bad. But I was crazy! They keep telling me I'm sick. I'm ill. Would he have exploded on a cancer patient for not following him? What if she yelled at him his whole shift? Would he have forcefully pinned a cancer patient down if she had to stop in the hall to puke instead of perfectly obeying his orders?"

He nods.

"I read this book, *The Crazy Game*, by Clint Malarchuk, the former NHL goalie. He made me realize that people with mental health problems say and do things without a filter. Lacking good judgment. I had no idea what I was saying. I just wanted out of that room. My actions were not intentional. I had no control. We went to the hospital for help. I needed help. They said they locked me up because they were concerned that I would be violent to myself or others, and then they watched me slam my head against the door without intervening. That guy needed to check his ego and show some compassion."

He nods again. Then he stands, moves to sit beside me, and takes my hand.

"So you think that's why they brought you the chair," Eric says.

I look at him with furrowed brows.

"Yes, so you would think they were treating me well."

"I talked to the people at the desk after that. The security guy was nice. He gave me a pamphlet with a number to call to complain. He was really helpful."

Of course he was. Doesn't Eric see the wool being pulled over his eyes? If I'm legit crazy and the staff are nice to him, why would he, or anyone, ever believe my accusations?

"You got really angry at me after that," he says. "They told me it would be better if I left because you were getting so agitated."

"I was agitated because I was alone and I never knew where you were and they were so mean and you were being so nice to them. Why would you leave when I needed you? Why would you do anything they suggested? That played right into their agenda."

"Reese, I don't think they had an agenda."

Sure, giving me a chair after assaulting me doesn't imply any kind of agenda. Especially when up until that point all they'd done was take things away to punish me. I bet they have an excuse for that too, like I could have used my magazine to strangle somebody or myself.

"I get that mistakes happen. I get that he probably didn't mean to do it. And maybe they didn't mean to lock me up like an animal or a prisoner and make things so much worse. But they did, so they need to be accountable. And they need to be taught how to do better."

I'm tired of this conversation and emotionally drained. Reliving it is too much. I know nobody will believe me, a middle-aged, unemployed, bipolar woman—the butt of a comedian's jokes. If they have no problem treating me this way, how are they treating other, less privileged, mental health patients? Or anyone without a lawyer husband? It must be fucking awful.

"So, we keep fighting," Eric says.

I smile a sad smile.

"And we get that apology," he continues.

I rest my head on his shoulder.

"And the hospital learns that staff need better training to work with mental patients. Especially the security guards."

"The whole world needs to learn that," I say.

He laughs. I'm not joking. Nothing about this is funny.

He wraps one arm around me.

"We'll save that battle for another day, okay?"

I nod, lean into him more.

"Thanks," I whisper. It's the best feeling in the world to know that Eric's got my back.

## 41. The New Doc

This office is calming. It has a wall of windows and even though today is a grey November day, the room is quite bright. The corner chair I sit in is comfortable without being too soft. My new psychiatrist's diplomas hang high on a wall, which seems humble. He has few personal effects on display, but there are some items that reveal who he is outside of this hospital. His bike helmet. His teapot. The framed picture of a tulip bed, which is propped sideways beside a collection of clinical tomes on his bookshelf. I'd like to ask him about it but we've only had a few appointments and I'm not ready to reveal my curiosity about the intriguing little things, or about art, or about his socks. He is stylish but not attention-seeking. Everything is professional and slightly muted, except for his colourful socks. They make me smile. They make me want to pay attention to my socks too.

Dr. Gordon offers me a coat hook but I decline. I'm already sitting on my coat and it makes me taller. I rearrange the shopping bags at my feet self-consciously. This hospital is downtown, close to many stores, so I always arrive early for pre-appointment shopping. Today I bought myself a pair of ankle boots. There is an Indigo nearby and I often have birthday gift cards in my purse, so I also buy the kids a treat. I find these rituals comforting—I'm not just visiting the hospital to see my shrink—but I guess they could be interpreted as overspending. Or lack of judgment, desire for instant gratification, and persuasive over-justification. Do ankle boots suggest hypersexuality? They do look good.

"Are you still riding your bike to work?" I nod towards Dr. Gordon's helmet.

I like inquiring about my support team during appointments. It pleases me when they share personal anecdotes. I know their time is precious and I don't want to waste it, but I like it when it feels like we're friends. I feel less like I'm greedily demanding their attention without offering mine in return. We're more on equal terms.

"Yes, I have been," he says and smiles. Encouraged, I tell him about when I used to build robots at University and King, and commute by bike from Yonge and Lawrence.

"It was the best. But I stopped in October when it got windy."

He talks about riding through the cold and we share a smile.

"So, Charise, how are you doing?"

How am I doing? I think I'm fine. I think I'm good. November always sucks because it's so dreary and an ominous reminder of the cold and drudgery to come, but somehow this November doesn't feel so bad.

"Good, thanks. I usually feel gloomy this time of year, but my therapist suggested planning small celebrations through November for fun."

"And it's working?"

"So far," I say.

"And what kind of things are you doing?"

"Little things. A pedicure. Gratitude notes. Ordering dinner when I'd normally cook."

He nods.

"That sounds good. And how is your sleep?"

I want to inhale deeply and release a big plume of air in one grand exhale, like a balloon being let go before the end is tied in a knot. I'm tired of talking about sleep.

"It's okay. I'll have a good night and then a bad night. And then another good night."

"And what do you do if you can't fall asleep right away? Do you start to feel anxious?" He speaks precisely, taking the time to choose each word carefully, so he says exactly what he means. The result is a slower-paced conversation than I have with most people, when we're both trying to squeeze in everything of importance. I like my conversations with Dr. Gordon. He is a good listener and makes me feel unhurried, so I take my time to express myself properly. He makes me feel important when we speak. Valued.

"No. I remind myself that it's just one night. I slept well enough the night before and a bad sleep tonight means I'll sleep better tomorrow. If I feel frustrated, I get out of bed, have a clonazepam, read, and turn on an audiobook or sleep app when I'm ready to try again."

"And that works?"

I nod. So far, so good.

"I like how you tell yourself that it's just one night," he says. "That's a good perspective to keep so you don't start to panic."

I agree. It's nice to feel a pat on the back, nice to hear I'm doing something right.

"It's a great way to frame it. It's a really good perspective."

His enthusiastic approval is encouraging.

"It's strange," I say, "I have a routine before bed. If I look at my phone or do anything requiring concentration, I'm too wired to sleep. It's like my brain can't handle thinking at night anymore. When I was in university, I used to study late into the night and then crash, and everything was fine."

"Yes, that's common." Dr. Gordon nods. "That sensitivity. It's like, you know, a Stradivarius violin. It's so sensitive because it's just so exquisite."

Did he really say that? Compare my brain with something exquisite? His smile suggests he's joking, but not in a way to mock or insult me. I feel his words. I feel their truth. I feel exquisite. No one has come close to describing my mental health, framing my illness, in a positive light. No one has tried.

"Let's look at your bloodwork," he says. He turns to his computer, pulls up my file, and checks my recent lab results.

"Everything looks better. Your numbers are well within range now. It's so strange that you weren't nauseous."

I was extremely lucky to find a family doctor, therapist, and psychiatrist within a few months of moving to Ontario. In our first appointment, Dr. Gordon detected that the lithium levels in my blood were too high, high enough to be toxic. He was surprised I wasn't vomiting. It surprised me too, because I am overly sensitive to everything but here I was, not sensitive at all to poison coursing through my body. I found the irony entertaining.

"That's good," I say. "I don't feel nauseous. But, I didn't then either."

Dr. Gordon dropped my dosage back to 900mg, from the 1200mg I'd been taking since May to overcompensate for the few weeks I took only 600mg. I guess it worked. I don't like to think about how sick I could have become had I stayed on a waiting list for a psychiatrist while continuing the 1200mg dose.

He asks about my job search, which I'm half-heartedly performing without enthusiasm or optimism since I've been unemployed for three years.

"I need to find something, it's just hard to make the right connection."

"Well, you are dealing with a lot right now," he says. "It could be very stressful."

This is true, of course, and clearly I don't handle stress well. But I also don't handle not working well.

"I think part of the reason I went manic in Alberta was because I wasn't working. I think if I had been there would have been other stress, but I would have had enough social support to cope. I don't think I would have been hospitalized or diagnosed as bipolar if I'd had a job."

Dr. Gordon looks at me without reacting. Then he tilts his head.

"Is that right?" I don't know if he's curious, finds this credible, or is simply humouring me because it's a ludicrous theory.

"I think so," I say with a shrug. I love being home with my children. But the menial tasks become so tedious, especially in a new city with no friends and few adult social interactions. "Who knows." It's all speculation.

"Make sure you keep drinking enough water going into winter. Many bipolar people don't realize how dehydrated they are and this affects medication."

I'm one of them. Maybe Dr. Patel told me to stay hydrated, like he patiently told me so many things, but if he did, it got lost in all that initial noise. Like the detail about synthroid and dairy. Or wine before pills, which I learned the hard way when I once took my lithium at my scheduled time, nine o'clock, and then went to a party. Or many little things that were never fully explained or if they were, it was when I was still too manic to comprehend or remember.

"That's good to know," I say. "Thanks Dr. Gordon."

Before catching the subway to head home, I detour to the art gallery on the hospital's main floor. Similar to pre-appointment shopping, this post-appointment ritual has become part of my routine. A way to process our conversation before turning my mind back to daily tasks. A way to take a calming moment for myself.

I don't fully understand these sculptures, but I appreciate them. A few pieces speak to me. The female warrior/mother. The trio that remind me of my children. The hard, strong protector. I sit in one of the comfortable chairs and admire the surroundings while making notes to remember specific details. Drink water. Lithium 900mg. Bloodwork three days before next appointment. Stradivarius. I won't forget Dr. Gordon's joke, but I write it down as an intentional reminder. To purposefully feel like I am special, instead of diseased. I am in a club with many amazing people. I might go out of tune, but I can be restored with the right help. I am exquisite.

## 42. Game Plan

"So, how's your sleep these days?"

I look up from post-dinner kitchen cleanup. It's January and we've been in our home for five months. Eric's question sounds innocent, but we both know it's not. The new year reminds us that spring will soon be here, and with it, fluctuating emotions that could lead to extreme mood swings and another manic episode.

"Okay," I say slowly. He waits.

"It's not great," I confess.

"It sounded like you were up a lot last night."

I'm surprised he noticed. He falls asleep fast and hard.

"I needed the bathroom. Then Jack was coughing. Then I was thirsty. Finally I went to take a sleeping pill."

I don't love clonazepam. It's always my last resort. But I use it when I know I should, when counting sheep becomes frustrating. Both manic episodes started with tossing and turning.

Eric is still watching me. Still waiting.

"I think part of the reason for my troubled sleep is because I'm getting anxious about going manic again in May." Christmas is barely over and I'm already starting to stress about spring. I really don't want a threepeat. I don't want to miss another Mother's Day.

He nods.

"One thing I've read about anxiety is that you have to think through the worst-case scenarios. So I've been thinking through them to figure out what I'm most afraid of."

"Good. What have you come up with?"

"The first is messing up Mother's Day again. For me, selfishly, but also for the kids, who spend a lot of time making crafts and get excited. So, to help with that, I wanted to ask if we can celebrate Mother's Day on another day, like whatever Sunday after I'm released from the hospital if I screw up again."

"Ok. What else?"

"The second is messing things up between us because I convince you to do something sexual that we regret." I know how persuasive I can be whether manic or not, but I also know that Eric knows my limits, and I trust that he would not let himself be convinced to break them no matter how tempted. He is my rock. But still, I feel the need to say this, to get it off my chest, to lighten the load I insist on carrying.

"That's fair. You know, you might do something you'll regret without me involved. How do we avoid that?"

I don't think that'll happen.

"Maybe. I haven't wanted to the last two times."

"You're very friendly when you're manic. It could easily be misinterpreted and one thing could lead to another."

We talk through scenarios and try to come up with solutions to potential problems. Our main solution is that I should avoid tempting situations altogether. Don't be alone with any man other than my husband or psychiatrist. No alcohol. I can handle that.

"Anything else?"

"Yes." I take a breath. "I'm afraid of two things in the hospital. Being locked up again and this time being forced into electroshock therapy."

"But you know they can't do that, right?"

"No. I don't think they can, but I don't know it. I still don't get what that form was about in Calgary and it said something about it being at their discretion to lock me up for thirty days. And then what? Can they just roll over into a new thirty days?"

"But you know I wouldn't let them, right?"

"I know you'd fight. But that doesn't mean you'd win against an antiquated medical and legal system. And what happens to me in the meantime? It would take ages."

"Well, I don't think they could give you electroshock therapy against your will. I don't even think they do that anymore."

"They do. In Calgary and Toronto."

He pulls his head back like a turtle.

"Really?"

I nod.

"Surely they need your permission. Or my permission."

"I don't know." I shrug. "That's my point. I think that form gave them permission to do whatever they decided was best. I just don't know. I don't even know if Ontario uses the same form as Alberta or if it's something more confusing that gives them more power."

Eric inhales and does a big exhale.

"So, what's the solution? What do we do if it happens?"

I look at him but stay silent. I have no solution if this happens. There is no light at the end of this tunnel. I won't be able to advocate for myself once I'm in the psych ward, because no one will listen to me, and we know from how I was treated last time that Eric will be powerless. They will tell him whatever they want and he will do whatever he thinks is best for me, which will be based on what they tell him. Even though we are now in Ontario and the hospital systems are different, neither of us know whether that is better or worse. Once hospital staff see that I've had two manic episodes, that crazy label will be firmly affixed if it wasn't already. I'm filled with dread as to how bad the third time could be considering how bad the second time was.

"I don't know," I say. "I guess we'll survive." Somehow.

"You should ask your doctor if they can do those things."

"Yes." But if I ask too many questions, will I seem too paranoid or untrusting? Will that trigger alarm bells? Will he make a note in my file?

I step forward, towards the hall. It's getting late and I need to start my bedtime routine. A shower, tea, yoga, TV, gratitude journal, reading that is neither too interesting nor too boring so my mind stays engaged but not excited, and lights out. It takes two hours but as I've learned the hard way, each step is critical. My calming routine is more detailed and specific than a baby undergoing sleep-training.

Eric reaches for me, pulls me close, and wraps his arms around me.

"I love you," he whispers.

"I love you too."

"I love all of you," he says. He pulls his head back to look at me before kissing me gently on the forehead.

He's said this before, that he loves all of me. I know he means well. I know his intentions are good. But it stings. It feels like I'm so fucked up, such a disaster, but he finds a way to see through my ugliness and love me anyway, and I should feel grateful. I've got my problems, sure, but so does he. So does everyone. I've also got a lot of things going for me, and I'm basically the same smart, beautiful woman he fell in love with twenty years ago. I want to tell him this, that I'm not a charity case, but we're sharing this nice moment and I don't want to wreck it. I don't think he'd buy it anyway, my argument that aside from future uncertainty, being bipolar doesn't feel like that big a deal anymore. That it's proving to be manageable if I stay structured, take my medication, and check in regularly with my psychiatrist and therapist. That episodes might happen but they can be treated fairly easily now that we know what to do, like diabetes. It's a condition, not a death sentence. There are positives about being bipolar, like my creativity, passion, and sensitivity, which help me to be a better mother, wife, and person. The sex alone is mind-blowing, even when I'm not manic. I'm pretty sure Eric wouldn't want to give that up. I'm pretty sure he's overlooking the good that comes with the bad when he says he loves all of me. I sometimes feel sorry for people who are not bipolar, those stable, perfectly balanced human beings who rarely experience true joy. True sorrow, yes, that comes with the territory. But true bliss. What a dream. It is like when Joe Banks abandons mediocrity to pursue passion in *Joe Versus the Volcano*, and ends up with enlightened happiness. It is surreal.

"I love all of you too," I say, a little sharp and a little cold. He's got issues, just like everybody. But there's no stigma attached to them, nor is anyone watching and judging his every move. He's not a freakshow like me. He hasn't been pigeonholed as unbalanced, incompetent, violent, or dangerous. There is so much misinformation and ignorance to overcome before society is no longer afraid of people like me. Is willing to believe people like me. Is willing to help people like me. This fight is daunting, but I can work slowly, one person at a time, starting with my husband. Just not tonight. Tonight it's late, and I have to wind down. I have to calm my mind. Tonight, and every night, I have to prioritize sleep. There will be no way to win this fight if I don't sleep.

## 43. Hypomania?

The trees are dancing again. Winter is slowly coming to an end and the trees are celebrating. This winter has been dark, gloomy, as winter is. It's only March, but already the temperatures are improving, the sky is blue instead of grey, and snow has melted to reveal vibrant green grass. The colours are impossible to ignore, and the universe has started talking to me again. Little things, like each light turning green as I drive up to an intersection, or a dog's warning bark when I'm about to step off a curb. I usually notice little things, but right now I notice them all. I certainly notice the men, their admiring looks and lingering eye contact. Maybe it's just spring fever. I don't think so though.

Traffic is heavy today. It's usually a fifteen minute drive to see Emma, my therapist, or as the title on her card says, Psychological Associate, but it's already been longer and I'm not there yet. I'll be late. I wasn't prepared for road construction season yet, it still feels too much like winter. The hard hats and dump trucks have recently appeared, much like the signs of possible mania, a little earlier than I'd expected. I call to mind Suzie's Good Days and Bad Days calendar and renew my internal resolve: *I will not go manic this spring.*

Emma stares at me, not unkindly, but uncomfortably. Like I'm here for observation, which I am, but it's more than that. I play with my braid to temper my nerves. I did my hair quickly this morning before noticing what I was doing. After realizing that this is the first time I've styled it in a braid since last May, I considered brushing it out. I would have if I hadn't been pressed for time.

"I've noticed my senses are keener lately, like they were before the two manic episodes," I say. Emma is often silent to encourage me to speak.

"Oh? How so?" She looks at me with caring eyes. Her face is kind and thoughtful, and when we hit on an easy topic the connection allows her to relax and drop her serious, professional mask.

"Everything is brighter." I wave a hand towards the blue sky outside her large window. "Moisturizer tingles when I put it on, like my skin is alive. Food tastes differently because my taste buds feel awake. My sense of smell is stronger. I often smell when dinner is ready right before it's about to burn."

"That must be helpful." She smiles.

"It is! I never have to set the timer," I smile back. "Music comes more naturally too. I can play the piano better, sing better, and hear the overlaps between songs all the time."

"Overlaps?" Emma squints her eyes and tilts her head, prompting me to explain.

"When two songs have the same chords. The newer one was maybe inspired by the older one. Or stole it."

"Can you give me an example?"

"Sure," I think for a moment. "Madonna's 'Express Yourself' and 'Born This Way' by Lady Gaga."

She smiles flatly. "I'll have to listen to them."

"It's okay," I say. "I'm also mixing food again."

"What do you mean?" Emma says.

"I spear a bite of something like, say pork. Then I dip it in mashed potatoes. Then I add a smear of peas or whatever vegetables we're eating."

"And then you eat it?" she asks. I nod.

"How does it taste?"

"Good. Better than separate." I think of the scene in *Ratatouille* where Remy teaches his brother how to mix food and every bite is an explosion of delight. Mine aren't fireworks but they're tasty.

"It doesn't sound like mania per se. Do you ever notice these things happening during the rest of the year, when your anxiety about going manic is not so heightened?"

"Sometimes," I say. I look at the ceiling to consider my response, knowing that Emma will wait patiently. "I think I notice these things at other times if I'm in a good mood and life is good. But when the snow melts and flowers appear, it's like I come alive again. It's like I fall asleep when summer ends, so I don't remember to mix food or pay attention to taste or smell or sound. And then spring arrives and I wake up and remember, or my subconscious wakes up and remembers, that my ideas were good and I should do them again. I'm suddenly more aware, which is great because I enjoy life more, but it's also scary, because I don't know if I'll get carried away again and enjoy life too much. The high is just really great. So it's tempting. People take a lot of drugs and pay a lot of money to experience a high I get from mania."

Emma laughs, but she knows I'm right. If big pharma could create a legal pill that brought on good mania symptoms and none of the bad, they would do it in a heartbeat. Even for the hypersexuality alone. Emma looks sympathetic. She has never been judgmental of anything I've told her, and I've told her a lot. She makes it easy to open up. I feel supported here.

"I think you hit on a good point, that sometimes during the rest of the year you might not be paying attention. These things might happen at other times, but since spring is traditionally when you've been manic, you look for any sign of mania in the spring. You're more likely to notice things that might be symptoms, because you had the same thoughts and behaviours last spring. It's good to know they might not all be symptoms of mania, because certain things do happen in spring that make everyone feel 'high'."

I nod and think of the colours, one of my early indications that mania might be lurking around the corner. This past winter was dreary, a combination of grey skies and white or dirty white snow-covered ground. When the snow melted and we finally saw the sun, the green grass and blue skies of course seemed bright by comparison.

"Do you notice any differences between now and the buildup to the previous manic episodes?"

I pause to reflect. This is a good question.

"Yes, three differences. First, even though the trees are bright, they don't glow. Last time everything had an aura and it started with the trees."

"Good," Emma says. "What else?"

"Second, I am still sleeping."

She nods. "And the third?"

"I can restrain myself from talking. The last two times I had to get it all out. Now, if I tell myself to keep my mouth shut, I actually do."

"Good. It's often helpful to focus on what is not the same to diminish anxiety that's building up because of similarities, which are more obvious."

Emma is a great therapist. She has more valuable insights than the nurse-therapist they assigned me as an outpatient back in Calgary, who was not a good listener. She kept checking her watch and we only ever discussed my diet and weight issues, which did not help me to accept or cope with my mental illness. I only saw her a handful of times before we both bailed.

"Charise, when you notice that your senses seem more awake, what do you do?"

I think before I reply. I spend half of our appointments together thinking. I like it that she never rushes me. I like trying to see where she's going and having time to look at something stale with her fresh perspective.

"Nothing. In my first mania I got excited. Each time I noticed something it felt like a sign from the universe. Now I try to ignore or downplay it."

"What do you do to downplay it?"

"I'll say to myself, 'Oh, yes, dinner's ready, the marinade smells strong tonight,' or, 'Jack dunks his pork in his soup and he's not crazy.' Anything to keep me from overthinking. Then I move on to something else."

"Like taking dinner out of the oven before it burns?" Emma smiles. I nod. "That's good you do that. There are some strategies you could try. We've talked about invoking an image or memory of someone or something that makes you feel the opposite emotion. So if you're feeling anxious you want to have an image on hand that will make you feel calm."

Sort of like Suzie and her Good/Bad calendar. That image makes me feel motivated. This makes sense. I have some memories that help me feel calm, like Nandy on her balcony, telling me her life story. Reading bedtime stories with the kids. My mom dabbing calamine lotion onto my chicken pox. My sister, marvelling at a double rainbow when we visited Banff. I feel better already.

"A second strategy is called five, four, three, two, one. Here, you want to purposefully label a number of items in your immediate surroundings that are associated with your senses. Five things you can see, four things you can feel, three things you can hear, two things you can taste, and one thing you can smell. This forces you into the moment."

Sounds hokey, but okay. I trust Emma. She's earned it. I ask about Cognitive Behavioural Therapy, which I would like to better understand, so we discuss it. Then we move on to meditation. Then somehow the conversation is back to what happened two years ago, when I went manic in May of 2017. When I made the garbage stew.

"Does anyone know what caused that first manic episode?" Emma says.

"Eric thinks it was because of my miscarriage. That I was triggered because it was spring. I kept talking about being pregnant and losing another baby. But I miscarried in 2005, and I dealt with my grief years ago. I don't think it's related."

She looks at me expectantly.

"The thing with me and babies in spring is that my miscarriage happened on May 3rd. So what would have been a joyful Mother's Day was instead a reminder that I'd failed. It hurt. The anniversary and tulips remind me, because I planted tulips as a memorial. Spring excites me because we've survived another winter and things grow from seemingly dead earth, but if something stressful like a move or vacation or frustrating job search makes me lose sleep, then my bipolar brain looks to the flowers, the babies, the pregnancies, the excitement for something hopeful. And the lack of sleep causes a tailspin and I might convince myself I'm pregnant. Or I've lost another one. Or both. Or something I don't know but it's baby related because my babies are what have given me my most joy and caused me my most pain."

She stays quiet. It's obvious that I now have a lot to say.

"I felt excited in 2017. A lot of good things were happening. I think I was also sad, because I had just turned forty and my little family was growing up. It hit me that I wouldn't have any more babies and my children didn't need me as much anymore. I think I struggled to accept that I'd never get to experience that baby bliss again. Never be needed like that again. I also missed Toronto. So, excitement combined with sadness combined with spring combined with loneliness combined with insomnia and total exhaustion." I shrug. I'm tired of talking, tired of overthinking something we'll never know for sure. We both sit silently, waiting for the other person to speak. Finally, she leans forward.

"How do you feel now about your miscarriage?" Her voice is probing but gentle.

"Fine," I say. Then I realize that might come across as harsh. "I mean, I'm not happy about it. But I don't ache like I used to. I wouldn't have Alex if I hadn't miscarried."

We share a moment of silence.

"I was thinking about volunteering with the support group that helped me grieve. But Eric and my sister aren't sure it's a good idea."

"Well," Emma says, "If you think you can talk about it without feeling affected then it could be great for you."

"That's what I think."

"Have you discussed it with your psychiatrist?"

"No, I'll ask him."

I'm buoyed by Emma's subtle reassurances and thank her as we wrap up. Before leaving the office, I stop to type a note into my phone so I'll remember: Does it happen the rest of the year too? When I start to worry that I'm shopping too much or am too sexual or irritable or creative, I will ask myself Emma's question. Our hope is that the hypomanic behaviour I'm concerned about in spring actually happens throughout the year, and I just don't notice because I'm not on high alert. I like this theory. I like many of Emma's theories. I'm lucky to have her, and my psychiatrist, and my family doctor, and my husband, and my children, and my parents, and my siblings, and my friends. It takes a village.

I pull my keys out of my purse and press the remote starter button for my minivan. It won't warm up in the time it takes me to cross the parking lot, but at least the heated seats and steering wheel will work faster. March is thawing out but to me it still feels freezing. Which is good. Too much spring weather too quickly could send me spiralling out of control.

## 44. Keeping the Lines Open

"Reese," Eric whispers. His body is draped across my legs, across our bed, in our dark bedroom. I groggily open my eyes.

"Yes?" I lift my head.

"Are you okay?"

"Yeah," I drop my head back onto the pillow. "What time is it?"

Andy Puddicombe's voice interrupts us as though to answer my question. The Headspace meditation app must still be playing on my phone, so it can't be much later than when I went to bed at eleven o'clock. Phew.

"Are the kids okay?" I ask.

"They're fine, everyone's fine. Go back to sleep."

He rubs my back. I close my eyes. I feel him stand and hear the floor creak as he walks away, and then I hear whispers from the hall. Pre-mania this would create a tidal wave of anxiety, but not tonight. I'm too tired.

"Morning," I say to Eric when he walks into the kitchen. I'm stirring the oatmeal in an attempt to cool it before I go wake the kids. Suzie doesn't like it hot. Mother's Day came and went without any fireworks this year. It was a relief for all of us that I was home and well. It was delightful to be celebrated without fear or anxiety, and I felt proud and grateful. I was also relieved when Sunday night rolled into Monday morning and I could put it out of my mind for another year.

"Morning." He hugs me. He holds me for a while until I break free to get back to breakfast. Today's a school day.

"How did you sleep?" Eric asks. He stays close, watching as I move between the counter, stovetop, refrigerator, and sink.

"Good, thanks. What happened? How come you woke me up?"

It is unheard of in our house for anyone to wake me up.

Before he can answer, Alex saunters into the kitchen rubbing his eyes. This is also unheard of. Alex is almost a teenager now, and he likes to stay up late and sleep in. Like me.

"Alex heard your podcast. It freaked him out."

I look to Alex as I place his bowl in front of him.

"It did? Sorry, Alex." I reach to stroke his hand as he picks up his spoon. He smiles.

"It's okay," he says. "I just didn't know what it was."

I have to get Jack and Suzie up but something tells me to stay here. I sit with my breakfast and start to eat. Eric joins us.

"Did it scare you?" I ask.

"Kind of," Alex says. "It had weird voices and sort of like chanting."

The voices I can explain. I don't know about any chanting.

"He asked me to check on you because he thought it was a mental health thing," Eric says, watching me closely. He wants to see if I will interpret my son's concern in a negative way and react badly. He says I overreact.

"Really?" I smile. It feels kind of funny. "It's just the podcast I listen to before bed. It helps me fall asleep."

"That's what Dad said." Alex smiles sheepishly.

"Thanks for looking out for me." I reach for his hand again. "Thanks both of you for looking out for me. I appreciate it." I smile at Eric, who smiles back.

"Appreciate what?" Jack asks, walking into the kitchen and sitting down.

"I appreciate you guys being so concerned about my mental health that you're always looking out for me." I lean in to hug Jack, and smile at Alex. I am so blessed.

"You know that day—," Alex says. We are watching television together after I've read a bedtime story to Suzie and Jack and kissed them both goodnight.

"What day?" I ask, probing because it irritates me when people don't finish their sentences, and I want to resolve it. I hang off of everybody's every word no matter what is being said. It is exhausting. I wish I could tune people out. Ignore the noise.

"You know that day we were in Edmonton," he pauses but this time I wait because we were rarely in Edmonton. After a moment he turns to me. "When you thought you were pregnant?"

I nod. I have vague, chilling memories of that manic trip home from Edmonton on Mother's Day of 2017. I remember excitedly, hysterically, sharing my news that they were going to have a new sibling. My mind spun this story and led me to believe it when I couldn't sleep in the Fantasyland hotel. I don't like to think about it. It makes me scared that I was so completely, illogically, insane, and it also makes me embarrassed. My young children must have been so bewildered. Dwelling on it won't provide any clues to prevent a reoccurrence. Better to focus on what I can control: sleep, drugs, diet, exercise, doctors, therapy. My healthy structured routine. This is what has prevented more manic episodes and it is all I can do. There is no cure. It's a lot to come to terms with. Even doing my absolute best, I might find myself back in the hospital next week, next year, or next decade, because there will always be factors that are out of my control—life events, aging, unexpected triggers. The good news, according to Dr. Gordon, is that my psychotic break reacted well to olanzapine twice before, so we can feel confident that it will work in the future. If I go manic again, we will deal with it. I trust him and my therapist, and I'm open with them about signs and symptoms. My family is learning what to look for, and we can talk about it. This team approach works with mental illness. Shame and stigma never help.

"Why did you think that?" Alex asks.

His seemingly simple question is actually quite complex. Does my son know the signs of pregnancy? We've been watching an episode of *Brooklyn Nine-Nine* where one of the characters is trying to get pregnant. Does Alex know what the test sticks are, and why she would only do them monthly? The show clearly prompted the conversation. Is he asking me a sex ed question, or, what I suspect is a more layered request to understand what was going on in my mind? I choose to follow my gut. He never asks me sex ed questions.

"That's a good question. When I told you guys, I hadn't taken a pregnancy test, but I'd been lying awake all night with my stomach churning. My period was late, so I convinced myself I was pregnant and far enough along to feel the baby kick."

"Why was your stomach churning?"

He must really want answers if he's asking for details.

"I'm not sure. Maybe dinner. So much food and it was all so rich, remember?"

He nods. I don't elaborate about the LED on the smoke detector in the hotel room, and how it randomly alternated between green and red, and started to flash at varying intervals. I don't tell him that in the darkness my vision and mind blurred until one LED became a pair of eyes that, combined with shadows, formed a dragon who revealed the certainty of the baby inside me by blinking in response to my yes or no questions. It didn't seem so bizarre at the time. Jesus, I was tired. And manic.

"Also, my period was late." I repeat my logical fallback explanation, the one that reassures me that I did have a credible symptom of pregnancy.

"So, you had reasons? Like, you actually believed you were pregnant?" Alex's facial expression is a mix of curious relief.

"Yes. I had reasons for everything I did, at least everything I remember. They always started out logical, even if my logic didn't make sense. I was so sleep deprived. Did you know sleep deprivation is a form of torture? It literally breaks people." He nods thoughtfully. He looks impressed, like instead of thinking of me as sick or weak, now I'm a survivor. More than that though, a fighter. Fierce. Strong. Maybe even a badass.

"Did Dad or I ever explain the symptoms of a manic episode?" I say.

"Well, like, I know you can't sleep. But you're not tired—you're really hyper. And you talk a lot, and sing. And you're really fun, like you let us eat more junk food and have more screen time." I suppress a smile, pleased by his description. It is bang on.

"Yup," I say. "I like the fun part a lot. I have really good memories of us having fun together before it got bad."

Alex nods.

"There are lots of symptoms, like 'delusions'. Me thinking I was pregnant is a delusion. I also convinced myself that those men in the mall parking lot were going to attack us or break into our truck. I could see it play out, like a movie, so I thought I could predict the future. Another symptom is poor judgment. A lot of manic people spend all their money on vacations or cars or anything that makes them feel good in the moment."

"Did you?"

"Hard to say. I splurged, but not in the same way. I justified everything as something I deserved, and they weren't big ticket items, so maybe I did. Like, I bought a purse for Mother's Day, but sometimes I buy myself a gift on special occasions. I kept putting junk food in the cart when Dad and I were grocery shopping. I wanted a bunch of expensive hair products at the salon." Memories of my excessive retail therapy keep popping up. "When I was going manic the second time, Dad and I went to Costco with a gift card to use up. It was exhilarating. I'd already started feeling some manic symptoms, and I wasn't far gone enough to ignore the warning signs, but I waved it off because Dad was with me. Like, if he approved of my behaviour I must still be okay." Or like an alcoholic who justifies a drink so long as he's not drinking alone. Somehow that makes things feel more under control.

Alex nods, paying close attention.

"Paranoia is another symptom, which is tricky." I wonder if I'm explaining too much, but Alex's body language prompts me to continue. "When I notice I'm hypomanic I wonder if I'm going manic or just paranoid that I might be. But if paranoia is a symptom, am I already manic? So I squash down my anxiety and tell myself I'm not paranoid. Then I can justify whatever I'm doing and tell myself I'm not going manic. Which might end up with me manic."

I can see by the look on his face that I lost him.

"Sounds confusing," Alex says.

"It is."

We stare at the television, which is now turned off. His head falls back to rest against the couch. I have more symptoms to describe but I don't want to overwhelm him.

"The most critical thing is sleep," I say. I need to get this last point across. "When I don't have enough or if I have too much, that's what makes me susceptible to mania or depression. You need a consistent healthy routine, but sleep is the key."

He's grown quiet. Contemplative. I reach out to touch his knee.

"You need to remember that," I say. "To prioritize sleep." Dr. Patel informed us that mental illness could be genetic, so it's always in the back of my mind. I don't want the kids to feel scared though. It's not the only contributing factor, and their awareness will help with prevention. "Everybody should prioritize sleep."

"I know," he says. He nods with a casual, almost dismissive, reassurance. Like he'll be okay whether he's inherited this disease or not. And he's right. He will be. I'm so proud of my self-assured soon-to-be teenager, and his younger siblings, who make my world so happy but also remind me to fight against too much happiness. To step back from temptation.

"Thanks for asking me about this, Alex. I hope my answer made sense."

"It did." He smiles.

"Thanks also for keeping an eye on me when you think my sleep is off, like when you told Dad about my podcast."

"No problem," he says. He makes it look easy. Like my mental illness is more of an inconvenience than an imposition. Maybe it is easy. Maybe we've made it easy. I wasn't sure where this conversation was going when we started, but my hope is that if we practice open communication our family will become more resilient for future challenges. Mental health problems are difficult at any age, so I want to plant as many prevention and coping strategy seeds as I can. Like many teenagers, Alex rarely expresses his thoughts or feelings to us, his parents, so any time he opens up we must pay attention. Talking together can only help.

# 45. Motherfuckers

"They are such liars! It's like they didn't even read my affidavit!" My hands shake as I flip through the letter from Alberta Health Services, scanning each page. I get to the end, which is a benign version of what I'd anticipated: "Based on the facts and evidence available to this investigation, there is nothing to support the initial allegation that Ms. Jewell was assaulted or that a CPO or SG used excessive force on her. As such, I am altering AHS' disposition of the issues identified in the original complaint from unfounded to unsubstantiated." To me this reads as: "The complaint you lodged against our protective services team member has been dismissed because you are crazy and delusional and nobody believes you, so you can go fuck yourself."

I turn back to the beginning. I'm tempted to take out a pen and write my comments and corrections directly on the paper, but this is the original copy. Despite my anger, I am sane enough to recognize that that is not a good idea.

Dr. Gordon and Emma would want me to calm down. I bring in a calming image. Nandy telling me a funny story. I take a breath, but I'm still holding the stupid letter and it still has control over me. I call in another image: Suzie, bedtime stories. It helps a little, but not enough.

"Eric!" I need to talk this out, but he doesn't reply. I call out again.

"They are such fucking liars! I didn't go into anybody's room. I talked from doorways to other patients who were bored and lonely and liked my company. Alberta Health Services even admitted I never went in, yet here they say I'm 'entering other patient's rooms?' And they never sent me pictures to identify the security guard, so how can they write, 'The Protective Services officer in which the complaint was made about,' if they don't know who it is? And they go on about trying to reach us but our phone numbers being out of service. I called them and changed the numbers and our address right after we moved. I spoke with that fucking bitch for half an hour to update everything. Somehow they managed to update our address but not our phone number? Super convenient."

I keep raging about the mistakes and blatant lies we've just received in this latest letter from AHS. The letter which will likely be the last, because we're at the end of the road. I don't want the stress anymore anyway. I have been friendly and cooperative from day one, over a year ago, and they continue to treat me like a lunatic who can't be tasked with handling her own affairs. Even this letter is addressed to Eric, even though it's regarding the complaint he made about my care while I was in the hospital, and even though we have both asked them to put me as the primary person of contact.

"Are you listening to me?" I say after I finish with the letter. I drop it on the countertop, resisting my urge to tear it into shreds. That, too, would be a mistake.

Eric walks into the kitchen.

"Yes, I heard." His voice sounds too hard. "I haven't had a chance to read it yet."

I can't control the look of anger on my face. It's not because of him. I'm not angry at him. I don't know whether he knows that.

"I'm going for a run." My outfit is not ideal but it'll have to do because I have to leave right now. This second. I lace up my shoes, grab my phone, and go, slamming the door on my way out.

"How was it?" Eric asks, walking into the backyard. When I got home I still craved fresh air, so I brought my yoga mat out to stretch.

"Great." My tone is flat.

"Oh. Was it not good?"

I glance at him, finish my downward dog, and sit cross-legged on the deck. How is it that this man who has loved me for so long still misunderstands me? My response was short because of anger, not sarcasm.

"No, it was great. Really great. It was hard."

This is the truth. I've been doing CBT thought records and mindfulness techniques to calm down but right now they feel like bullshit. Running hard helped more.

"So, I read the letter properly."

He reaches for my hand, and I allow myself to be pulled up and led to the couch. I don't care where we have this conversation. Comfort won't make what he's about to say less disappointing. I'm not angry at him. I'm just not stupid and it's easy to see the writing on the wall. I don't need to be placated.

"They lied," I say before letting him speak. I want to be on the record first. "They said things that did not happen or contradicted things they've said before. They said there's no evidence when we all know there was a camera in that room 'for my protection.' So, what? They turn the camera off when it's convenient? Like, as soon as one of their people go into a patient's room and they don't want evidence? Or, what? They delete the recordings as soon as a complaint is filed? They are fucking liars."

Eric reaches to stroke my back. I prop my head on my hands and sit hunched on my knees at the edge of the couch. I breathe. The hospital is a place where sick people go to get better. Where staff are supposedly so trustworthy that they declare anyone who doesn't immediately trust them to be paranoid. Not a place for staff who can't control their tempers to physically assault women half their size, women who are there for help. Since the moment Eric filed the complaint, the only things I've requested are an apology from the Peace Officer or Security Guard or Protective Services whatever the fuck label they want to give him, an apology from the nurse who denied my bathroom requests, and to improve training or procedures to prevent such occurrences from happening in the future. Training regularly needs improvement, especially in a field like Mental Health. Why is Alberta Health Services more concerned about protecting their staff than resolving problems to protect their patients?

"I know, shhh." Eric's voice is soothing, not condescending. He pulls me towards him and I rest my head on his chest. And then he starts to talk. About the next steps for the complaint, filing criminal charges, travelling back and forth during a trial, stuff we both know is not going to happen. I'm not going back to Alberta to fight a losing battle in a court room. It's not worth the exorbitant amount of money it will cost us, or the frustration I will feel every time I am treated like a crazy person. I need to protect my mental health, which means reducing stress.

"If you want, we'll do it," he says. "I'll figure out the law. I'll go out there to fight. We'll take it as far as we can. We'll mortgage the house if we have to."

I know he means it.

"No, it's done. It's their word against mine and I'm bipolar. I have no credibility. No one will believe me."

He rests his chin on my head and slowly strokes my upper arm.

"We can do it if you want. We can try if it will help you."

"It was never about helping me. It was about recognition for better treatment. Who else has this happened to?" A single tear rolls down my cheek. Eric leans over and kisses it so tenderly that I barely feel his lips. Then he wraps both arms around me and we slouch down into the couch. We stay this way for a while, listening to the cicadas. I could fall asleep on his chest in this backyard, but one of the kids calls from the house so it's time to go in. It's time to accept that it's over. I know what happened. I've spent enough time doubting myself since my diagnosis when I lost all self-esteem, and I'm not doing it again. I know what happened. Those assholes, and the assholes who are covering up for them know what happened too. Someday it'll catch up to them. Someday the karma train will run over

ALL the assholes who deserve it. For my own well-being, I decide to let the universe handle them and not rely on the healthcare or justice systems. I decide to let go of waiting for an apology for the past and put my energy into change for the future. I just don't know how I will do that.

# 46. Killing them Softly

I feel low. Lower than after my first mania. I know my memory is correct. I know the assault happened. I know I am in the right and they are in the wrong. But even though I know this, their refusal to admit their wrongdoings has caused me to spiral into numbness. The weight of it and not knowing what to do with it is heavy. It's causing melancholy, depression. I feel small. No grandiosity now.

"Why are you crying, Momma?" Suzie says as she walks into the room. Her room, the one she shares with Jack, where I'm lying in Jack's bed. It's my safe space. Nothing bad has ever happened to me here. She sits down and nestles into me.

"I'm sad." I wrap one arm around her. I rest my hand on her head and gently stroke her hair.

"What's wrong?" she says. She reaches to hold my hand. My seven year-old has more insight into people's moods, and how to help, than most adults I know.

"I don't think I'm doing a good job," I whisper. She looks at me, concerned. "I don't think I'm good enough to be your mom." Tears overflow as I say the words out loud. Words that up until now have only lived inside my head. Words that have only asserted themselves twice: once after my diagnosis and now, after being betrayed by the Alberta Health System.

"Sweetie," I say, shifting position to maintain eye contact. "I think I have to go away." My words are intentionally vague, because I don't know exactly what I mean. All I know is that they deserve a better mom. All I know is that they deserve more.

"No!" she insists, her little hand grabs mine and her arm pins me to the bed. Then she jumps up and runs to the door.

"Jack!" she calls down the hallway. And again, "Jack!"

She must see him approach, because she rushes back to lie with me, as though afraid that I'll leave if she doesn't. Jack walks into the room as Suzie cuddles into me.

"Yeah?" Jack asks. He smiles, always happy to be needed.

"Mommy wants to go away!" Suzie says, her voice full of emotion.

"No, sweetie, I don't want to." I kiss her forehead. "I just think I should. I think you guys need a better mommy."

Jack walks across the room to sit with us.

"Oh," he says. He clucks his tongue and shakes his head. "No." He has the relaxed confidence of someone who knows all the answers. He has the relaxed confidence of his father. But they don't know all the answers. They don't even know all the questions. Still, his calm demeanour is reassuring.

"Where would we get a better mommy?" Suzie asks. The hopelessness in her voice forces me into this moment. What am I doing to my poor children? Why am I exposing them to my inner turmoil? No kidding they need a better mother.

"Daddy would find one," I say. She clings to me. "She'll make good food and play with you and do crafts."

"No. You're the best mommy," Jack says. He puts one hand on my forehead as though taking my temperature. "You're just a little tired."

I'm not ready to accept that I belong in this family, that I am worthy of these marvellous children, but his wisdom makes my heart smile. It is only because of them that I am still here, that I get out of bed every morning and go to bed every night, and that I can resist the dark voices that sometimes invade my mind and my heart and try to persuade my body to follow along with their terrible ideas. The term "bipolar" officially replaced the commonly known "manic-depressive" in 1980, for clarity of diagnosis and to reduce stigma. Mania is something I have only recently had trouble with. Depression has tormented me since I was a teenager. The worst episode followed my miscarriage—when I did consider ending my life—but I've had other dark times: homesickness in university, post-partum syndrome I mistook as baby blues, the failure of my one attempt at entrepreneurship. I read somewhere that suicide is the number one cause of death in bipolar people, which is terrifying. Up until now my children have always brought me out of my lethargy and despair, but what if one day it's not enough? I have to believe that I will call on my psychiatrist and therapist and husband to support me if it ever gets that bad. I have to believe that I will ask for help.

"You're probably right, Jack." I pull him down, and we lie together for a while.

"Did you draw that star, Jack?" Suzie asks. Jack and Suzie share a bunkbed with Suzie on the top, so the underside of her bed is his ceiling. I sometimes lie in Jack's bed for a pick-me-up, and draw a little doodle on the wooden frame above his head. I like gifting surprises.

"What star?" Jack says. Suzie points to show him. It's the first time he's noticed it, even though he sleeps below it every night. Relaxed confidence, but not the most observant. Just like his father.

"I drew it," I say.

"You did?" they ask in unison. I nod.

"I thought you might see it and smile."

They both hurry to tell me how much they like it, and then move on to pointing out some of my other little doodles.

"Can we draw on furniture?" Jack asks.

"Sometimes," I say. "Do you remember when we moved and each of you drew on the bottom of a drawer?"

They look at me with blank faces.

"You were little. We'll pull them out some time so you can see. It was great. You created secret art. Nobody knows about them. There's something I love about drawing in a hidden space. I guess I just love surprises." Likely because my mom was so good at them.

"But this isn't really hidden," Jack says. "It's on the bottom of the bunk. Anyone could see." He's right, of course. He usually is.

"True, but it's not obvious," I say. "You didn't see it. It's subtle."

They nod in a way that makes them look wise. I think I'm the only one who remembers the first half of our conversation. While I still think it's true, they'd be better off without me, the intensity of the feeling has subsided. I can choose to ignore that voice, at least for tonight. I can choose to move on. At least for right now. *This too shall pass.*

# 47. Misunderstandings

Eric walks into the family room and sits down. I glance at him then return to the screen. The credits start to roll, so I reach for the remote. He turns to me.

"I think we should talk about what to do if you go manic again."

I am not expecting this. Eric rarely initiates a conversation about mental health, or anything heavy that could turn tense. Also, it's fall. It's been a year and a half since my last manic episode, so to me it feels like we're out of the woods, or at least in the calm before the next spring storm. I guess he wants to discuss it when I'm less anxious.

"What do you think we should do?" I say, turning the television off.

"I don't know. That's why I'm asking you."

I'm pleasantly surprised. I like being trusted. I like feeling like I'm the expert of myself.

"Do you remember what to watch out for?" We've discussed it many times, and Eric has accompanied me to psychiatric appointments where he made detailed notes on his phone. I'm not sure he remembers the specifics, but it's all written down.

"If you're not sleeping, talking fast, argumentative." He looks up at the ceiling. "If you're hypersexual."

"Yes. Also I become obsessed with colour and nature. Everything becomes art, remember? Even garbage is beautiful."

I start to list more symptoms: I'll repeat myself because I can't focus long enough to know I'm repeating myself. My senses are razor sharp. I constantly talk about song similarities or an apple's delicious sweetness. I want tea all the time, mostly for the heat and aroma. I multitask to the extreme and become hyper productive. I tune out when bored with conversations and then tune back in based on tone and pauses, so I can ask meaningful questions. This way I have one ear on the kids, a mundane task, or I can focus on the beauty of nature, while still appearing to be a good listener who is paying full attention.

"Right." He nods slowly.

"In the first mania, I became consumed by travel and religion, so that could happen again," I say. "And I want to help everyone. Everybody becomes a charity."

"Yes. You started giving all our stuff away last time."

"I did, but that was also to sell our house and move. And it was stuff we didn't need."

He gives me a look, like, "Don't push that button." I remember what I gave away. It was stuff we didn't need.

"And I have a lot of ideas," I say. "Most of my sentences start with 'We should.'"

"Right, I remember that." Eric says.

"Everything I do is more confident. I sing louder, I workout harder, I talk to myself to walk through whatever I'm doing. I don't hesitate."

"Okay," he says. "But if those signs start appearing, what do we do?"

I think we've had this conversation before, but it's worth repeating. I'm glad he's asking.

"Before it gets bad, what I need is truth and kindness. The kids know what's going on and if we sugarcoat it that makes them confused, which confuses me. Also, if nobody tells me they're worried then I think I must be fine, because nobody's worried."

"I'll tell you when I notice the signs."

"I don't know if you will. The last time I felt like I might be hypomanic I told you and you said you'd already noticed. I don't know if you didn't want to freak me out or were hoping it would pass or just didn't want to talk about it."

My tone is gentle, because I am not trying to be accusatory. Eric took excellent care of me. I watch as he inhales and exhales through his nose. His mouth is clenched as tightly as his fists.

"Okay. Truth and kindness. Got it."

"You know when you made plans for me with my friends—when you needed a break?"

He nods.

"That was great. Every time I was with someone new it felt comforting."

His face contorts like I just slapped him. I don't know why at first, but then I realize.

"That's not what I meant. I felt comforted by you too." Except when you were angry, I think but don't say. I know he did his best. Nobody is comforting when they're angry. "Comfort from a friend, especially those women, is different. They just let me talk. They didn't say I needed rest, or tell me what to do. They just listened."

"Probably because they weren't with you all the time! You were exhausting!"

I wait to see if there's more, because he's giving me a look like he's holding back. But then he turns away.

"Probably," I say. "It was easy for them. That's why it was a great idea. It helped me, and gave you a break. Like grandparents."

He looks at me again. He looks tired. I want to support him for all he's been through, but I don't quite have it in me. I think it would help him to talk to a therapist, but I won't ask. There's enough tension already.

"If I go manic again, I think you should record me. I think I will be angry, and doubt you, so afterwards when I'm trying to remember everything and we're trying to pick up the pieces, it would help if I could listen to our conversations. To better understand and explain my motives."

"Okay. So, kindness, truth, friends, and record you. Anything else?" Eric says the words so abruptly that they sound cruel. His jaw is clenched.

"Why are you angry? What were you expecting when you started this conversation?"

"I'm not angry," he snaps. I raise my eyebrows.

"I'll need to call your mom." His tone is slightly softer.

I nod. That's a good idea. My mom is very kind.

"Do you remember we talked about having a mantra?" I ask. He nods.

"Dr. Gordon suggested we have a saying for if either of us suspect mania. Something that's unlikely to trigger anger on either side. He suggested 'The colours seem brighter.'"

"Okay," he says.

"Okay, like, you want to try it?"

"Sure." The word sounds like a shrug. He leans back against the couch and stares straight ahead. I want to ask if he remembers Dr. Gordon's instructions for clonazepam versus olanzapine if my insomnia starts again. Or if he can find his notes from that appointment on his phone. But he's too annoyed. I don't know why, if I've done something wrong again, but I know he won't tell me anything he doesn't want to. I don't see any point in continuing a one-way conversation, so I pick up the remote.

"I just don't want it to happen again," Eric says. His eyes are open wide, staring at the ceiling, and he turns to look at me. Look into me. He looks sad.

"Me neither," I say, taking his hand. "At least Dr. Gordon says that since olanzapine worked twice before it would likely work again for a manic episode."

He nods. I could keep trying to reassure him, but I don't know what the future holds. All I know is that we've got this moment, and this moment is pretty good. I lean back, into his chest, and turn on the TV. This moment is actually pretty great.

## 48. Stigma

November. Such a dreary month. A stop-gap between the beauty of October and the excitement of December. Melancholy typically sets in around now, but this year feels different. I am not low and I am not high. Neither catatonic nor inspired. I've been told this is how non-bipolar people feel on a regular basis. How boring.

Jack and I are the only ones remaining at the dining room table. He has a meal that he's diligently working away at. I have a glass of cabernet sauvignon that I'm savouring. Everyone else has scattered.

"Jack, do you remember 'The Garbage Tree?'" Jack is ten. I don't know how much he remembers from that fateful weekend two and a half years ago. He looks up, head snapping back, forehead furrowed.

"What garbage tree?" he says.

"The one I made on the wall in our Calgary house. On Mother's Day, when I was manic."

Jack nods.

"With the newspapers?"

"Yes—I made it while you guys watched *Inside Out*." I'd requested that movie for Eric to watch. The rest of us had already seen it. I thought he might learn something about emotions, like I did. I think it's brilliant.

"I remember," Jack says. "After Edmonton."

"Exactly. Do you remember what you thought it was?"

He chews, thoughtfully, before replying.

"Someone thought it was fire. I think someone thought it was an arrow. It was a tree?"

I nod. I'm impressed.

"You thought it was fire. Alex thought it was an arrow. We were all right."

"Oh," Jack stabs a potato and pops it in his mouth. "I liked it. What happened to it?"

"I don't know. It was gone when I got home from the hospital. I guess Daddy took it down." I guess he didn't like it.

"That's too bad."

We sit in silence. He finishes his last few bites and turns to me.

"Mommy," he pauses, looking over my shoulder to gather his thoughts. "Why do you call it that?"

I smile. This kid doesn't miss a thing.

"Because it was made of newspapers. Which I took from recycling, so I guess technically it's 'The Recycling Tree.'"

"Or, 'The Newspaper Tree.'"

"Yes. Or, 'The Newspaper Fire.'"

He leans in for a hug. I wrap my arms around his shoulders and he wraps his around my waist.

"You know what though, Jack?"

He looks up.

"I like my original name best, 'The Garbage Tree.'"

"Why?"

"I don't know. That's how I think of it. Because I made it to look like a tree, out of materials that had been discarded. I think that name has a nice ring."

"I guess. It sounds like garbage. So it should be thrown away."

"Well, it was thrown away."

He looks deeply into me. He does this to determine if I'm emotional. If I'm about to cry.

"Do you think it's a bad name?" I say.

"I don't know." Jack rarely doesn't know his thoughts. He does know that he doesn't want to hurt anybody or get into trouble.

"Do you know what a stigma is?"

He nods slowly. Even the word stigma sounds scary.

"Do you think garbage is bad?" I prod.

"Kind of. It's garbage."

"True. There's an expression, 'One man's garbage is another man's treasure.' Have you heard it?"

"Nope." He pulls away. I'm losing him.

"It means that something I discard might be valuable to you."

He pushes out his chair, stands, and picks up his dishes.

"It's just a name, Jack. A label. A label doesn't determine if something is good or bad. It only takes on value based on the meaning we assign it."

"Okay, thanks Mommy." He takes a few steps and then turns back. "Sorry it got thrown away."

I smile.

"That's okay, Jack. Thanks though."

He leaves me to my solitude. There is so much more I want to explain but I reassure myself that it will come with time. I've been labelled sensitive, intriguing, intense, thoughtful, kind, clever, emotional, unstable, unbalanced, bipolar, crazy, and a maniac. Sometimes these labels were complimentary, or factual. Other times they were hurled at me with the intention to harm. I used to cringe at certain words, like 'crazy,' or 'insane.' They bounce off my dragon skin now, like dull, useless arrows. Most of the time. They're just words, just like 'garbage'. Sometimes they're accurate, other times ignorant. I hope one day I can express this properly to my children. To reassure them that just because a stigma exists doesn't mean it deserves our attention. And to give them hope.

Our family has come a long way. I don't remember our early conversations about my diagnosis and mental health. Eric must have explained it to the kids while I was in the hospital, and then they didn't talk about it around me, believing that to be the best strategy. When life returned to semi-normal, I began to wonder why it was so taboo, even in our house. I knew they must have had questions about something so significant, and I was concerned that they were bottling up their emotions. I started to slip it into everyday conversations whenever I saw an opportunity, like when a song by Linkin Park came on the radio.

"Did I tell you about this lead singer, Chester Bennington?"

"Maybe," someone would say. They always wanted me to talk about him even after they remembered his story.

"He died by suicide. He was devastated after one of his best friends died and he couldn't find the help he needed."

"But he's such a good singer."

"I know. Even talented people face challenges. We all have to be able to talk about our feelings." I want my children to know that mental health is part of overall health. There should be no shame in asking for support

"Did he have kids?"

"He did. I think four or five."

"That's really sad."

"I agree."

At first my family resisted my initiatives, because they didn't want to connect the dots between me and sadness, let alone me and suicide. They didn't ask me questions, but the more I forced the conversation, the more they responded. I eventually did what I always do: borrowed library books so they could read someone else's words and it could open up a dialogue.

"This one's about a family of polar bears where the mom learns she's bipolar after a manic episode." I held up the book for them to see the picture on the cover.

"*The Bipolar Bear Family*," Jack read the title and then tilted his head. "She should have called it *Bearpolar*."

"Yes!" Suzie said. "They're polar bears!" She looked happy, delighted to get the joke.

To this day, over a year after I brought that book home, Jack still refers to it as *Bearpolar*. I love his adapted title. It speaks to strength, not weakness.

Once the books and conversations helped reduce the stigma in my own family, I began to discuss my mental health more openly with the outside world. Much like my Linkin Park segue into a conversation, I paid attention to opportunities and then leaped, albeit hesitantly in the beginning. The first time I shared my story with a stranger was about six months after my diagnosis. We were at a party, I'd had too much to drink, and it was hard to get the words out. I could have stayed quiet, but the woman I was talking to was discussing her background—clinical psychology—and her passion for mental health issues. Despite being tipsy I recognized it as a chance for me to open up, which I knew was necessary if I wanted to stop feeling ashamed. I told her my story as briefly as I could and ended with the words, "So it turns out I'm bipolar." I waited for her reaction with tears in my eyes: a combination of embarrassment and gratitude for her sympathetic ear. At first she seemed stunned, but she was so nice and curious and the more we talked, the more I settled down and began to feel comfortable. Since then I've forgotten how many people I've told. Some react with kindness or sympathy and others take it in stride and continue the conversation without missing a beat. It has occasionally been awkward, but I try not to take it personally.

"I don't know if you know, but I'm bipolar," I'll say to a new friend. There is not usually a reason why the person would know, but I've found this to be an effective way to slip it into a conversation rather than a direct, "I'm bipolar." It gives the other person an easy way out: "No, I didn't know," or "Yes, so-and-so mentioned it." It also lets me own my mental illness in a way that minimizes its significance, which is empowering. Every time I talk about it, the words become easier to say. I'm often complimented on my openness and willingness to be vulnerable, so much so that it no longer feels like a vulnerability.

My wineglass empty, I stand and carry the remaining dinner remnants from the table to the kitchen, forcing myself into the present moment. I don't want to sit in my wine buzz stupor thinking too hard in case I hit a nerve. Even one glass of wine can push me too high or too low if I let it, so I don't. I'd rather prevent a fire than have to put one out.

# 49. An Open Book

I am not a liar. It's not worth it. When I lied to Dr. Patel about my medication in 2018 I felt guilty, but not nearly as guilty as I felt keeping it a secret from Eric. I strive to be honest, especially about my mental health. Especially with my psychiatrist and husband. No white lies. No whoppers. No lies of omission. No secrets. Nothing. Truth and only truth. For this reason, I sometimes feel anxious before a psychiatrist's appointment. I'm not sure what I might reveal, and what it might say about me, let alone what the repercussions might be. But today, I don't feel anxious. Today, I feel eager, excited. Today's appointment is special.

Dr. Gordon looks happy to see me. He usually looks happy in the stressed, busy way of a good person who is making a difference, but today he is happy in an appreciative way, because today I am helping him instead of vice versa. I am here for an appointment at his request, for a resident to interview me as a calm, asymptomatic bipolar person. Apparently residents don't have much access to mentally ill people who are not in crisis, which could partially explain why patients are often misunderstood. If students only ever see us in crisis, that will always be the basis of their assumptions. A resident who only sees me at my worst might never consider that I have a "normal" side. Might never consider that I am not always angry and ugly, and that I'm worth trying to save. I'm worth compassion and respect, not restraints and abuse. I'm a human being.

When Dr. Gordon asked me to consider being interviewed to provide his resident with an opportunity to improve his skills, I immediately said yes. Anything that improves medical training will improve treatment. We are both happy to see each other.

The resident sits in Dr. Gordon's desk chair while Dr. Gordon is relegated to the corner. This resident is young, tall, and looks like someone I would picture working at Dunder Mifflin rather than training to become a psychiatrist. He stands, introduces himself as Dr. Howard, and thanks me for coming. We all sit. Dr. Gordon is here as a silent observer and will take notes about Dr. Howard's technique. He informs me that I don't have to answer anything I don't want to, so there is no reason to be nervous. I'm not nervous. I think it'll be fun.

The first questions are typical. My name, age, where I live, who I live with, and the like. Anything that might be considered sensitive is asked in a thoughtful way, to avoid any misinterpretation. So instead of saying, "What do you do?" or, "Do you have a job?" he asks, "How do you support yourself financially?" It's clever. Such a simple way to help a patient feel safe rather than small, because it can be hard to work with a mental illness but admitting unemployment can make us feel lazy and incapable, adding to our insecurities.

"Can you tell me how you arrived here?"

I'm not sure what he means. I took the subway. Does he want to know if I can drive?

"Like, arrived today?"

"No. How it is that you came to be here with Dr. Gordon?" He stumbles a bit, but he'd like me to explain my history and why I need a psychiatrist. I guess some patients might be sensitive to more direct questioning here too.

"Sure." I describe my first manic episode and hospitalization, my second manic episode and hospitalization, and our move to Toronto.

"And, how did you know you were having a manic episode the first time?" This question is a bit odd. Does anyone really know the first time?

"Well, I didn't, not really. My husband took me to the hospital because he didn't know what else to do."

"Right, but what was the first indication that something was off?"

"I served garbage for dinner."

We go through the details of the first mania. He then asks about the second mania. I openly admit that I self-reduced my lithium dosage. I've learned my lesson about withholding information. His eyebrows arch. He seems mildly surprised. I don't know if it's because of my disobedience or my honesty.

"Why did you do that?" he asks gently.

"I didn't like the side effects. I felt flat and foggy all the time." I imagine this is why most bipolar people stop taking their meds. A medicated life isn't horrible, but sometimes it's not a lot of fun.

"Have you ever had any issues while driving?"

"No." The first time I drove after being hospitalized was frightful. I was certain I would have an accident because my foggy mind wouldn't allow me to react quickly enough in traffic. Luckily everything went smoothly otherwise I'm not sure I would have regained the confidence to drive again.

"Nothing? No racing? No interactions with police?"

"No," I shake my head. He looks at me like he's trying to catch me in a lie. I don't know how else to deny something that never happened. "Nothing like that." His question makes me realize how many bipolar people must have those kinds of problems. How mental illness can be criminalized.

"Have you ever had any substance abuse problems?"

"No."

"Do you use any substances right now?"

No drugs, but what else could substances mean? Does an occasional cigarette count? Alex learnt that caffeine is a substance, so should I mention that?

"No."

"Nothing?"

"No."

"Marijuana? Heroin? Cocaine?"

What kind of middle-aged suburban stay-at-home mom-of-three does he think I am? It dawns on me that perhaps my experience being bipolar is vastly different from others'.

"No," I shake my head.

"Alcohol?"

"A glass of wine with dinner. My first psychiatrist approved this amount the first time I was discharged."

"Just one?"

"Yes, except socially. Dinners with extended family. Holidays."

"How much do you drink then?"

"Two glasses. Three at most, spaced out."

I explain that if I drink more I start to feel symptoms similar to extreme mood swings. Once I feel manic or depressed I no longer have enough awareness to cut myself off, and I won't listen to Eric if he suggests I stop.

"It sounds like you've really figured out your limits and have a good amount of self-control to stick to them," Dr. Howard says. He appears impressed, like this is not something a bipolar patient is typically capable of, which is not surprising if he only sees patients during extreme episodes. I've been given many compliments about my self-control, discipline, and personal awareness. It mostly feels like the key to controlling my disorder is simply structure. Sticking to a routine, doing the things everybody is supposed to do for optimal health, and taking medication to smooth out any kinks.

"My grandfather was an alcoholic. I know it's something I need to be aware of."

He prompts me to elaborate.

"Ideally, I think I shouldn't drink alcohol. But I am very structured and disciplined, and I have a limited diet already, so I want to hold onto one of my few remaining pleasures if I still feel in control and have no significant effects."

He nods again and a smile spreads across his face. He looks so encouraging, and also so young. I feel proud to help this man learn how to help people like me. I feel like I'm doing something meaningful.

"That makes sense to me," he says. "And what medication are you currently taking?"

I easily list them: lithium carbonate, synthroid, and occasionally clonazepam. But when he asks about dosages I smile and shrug. I tell him what I can. Lithium is 1050mg after some tweaking with Dr. Gordon, clonazepam is whatever I need it to be if I can't fall asleep, within limits I can't recall, and synthroid has stayed the same for almost three years and still I don't know. I'm not interested in wasting what little brain capability I have trying to remember drug dosages a doctor could learn from my file, my psychiatrist, my family doctor, or my pharmacist. There's enough redundancy there.

"Do you ever hear voices? Or have visions?"

I pause, because I'm reluctant to admit something that is so obviously 'insane'.

"Sometimes when I'm close to falling asleep I hear what sounds like my husband playing guitar. Or I think the TV is on. But when I check, the house is silent."

He nods. Writes something down that I would love to read. "That's what we call a hypnagogic hallucination. They're fairly common. It's not a symptom of bipolar, and not something to be concerned about."

Huh. I've been hearing these noises for at least a decade, and since my diagnosis they made me really stressed. Hearing them right before I'm about to fall asleep jars me awake and makes me anxious, which then prevents me from falling asleep. I thought they were a sure sign of my particular brand of crazy. In three sentences this doctor has removed all of that anxiety. Remarkable.

"Have you ever self-harmed?"

"No."

The conversation turns to suicide. If I've attempted it. If I've contemplated it. If I've ever made a plan. I reply with the truth: no, yes, yes. He takes my answers in stride, as though they are the most natural thing in the world. As though he's asking me if I've ever had coffee or contemplated having coffee or made a plan to have coffee.

"And so, what was your plan?"

The way he asks makes me think my answer should be easy.

"Well, I don't know if it was a plan. I didn't think it through in great detail. I just knew how I would go about it, generally."

He presses me further in a gentle but firm way, and I grudgingly answer his questions as vaguely as possible. This is uncharted territory for me in this calm, comforting office. I don't remember telling Dr. Gordon that I thought about suicide after my miscarriage. I might have and I've forgotten; we talk about many things. I glance at him to see if his face registers any surprise or disappointment, but it does not. He remains neutral. I feel ashamed.

Thankfully Dr. Howard ends that line of questioning. We discuss exercise and diet, and he again compliments me for my self-awareness and discipline. He then asks about my parents and childhood, and keeps rephrasing his questions as though looking for clues as to why I am the way I am. Which, I suppose, is exactly what he's doing, because there are links connecting childhood trauma to bipolar mood disorder. He won't find any answers in my happy childhood, my loving parents. We talk briefly about my South African past, siblings, and husband. He's trying to paint the whole picture, but with quick dabbing brushstrokes. He could use some precision. When he wraps up the interview, he asks for feedback. Anything I thought he should have asked to get to know more about me.

"Well, I mentioned my grandfather was an alcoholic. He was likely bipolar. I think it might have been worthwhile to talk more broadly about my family rather than focus so much on my parents."

Dr. Howard seems appreciative of this criticism. He adds a note to my file, thanks me, and stands to shake my hand. Dr. Gordon walks me out, we do a quick debrief, and he thanks me too, going so far as to give me a completely unnecessary card and gift. I should be the one giving him a gift, to thank him for making me feel valuable.

"I forgot you were from South Africa," he says. "We'll have to talk about that some time. I worked there for years."

We chat briefly, and it doesn't surprise me to learn that his work was humanitarian. I love that of everything I just spoke about, Dr. Gordon chooses to end today's meeting on a positive note. I feel relieved. Non-judged. This is a person I can trust. He's also someone who trusts me, and that feels best of all.

This will be the way forward.

# 50. Spiralling Out

I put on my boots, pull the laces taut and tie them at the top. We've almost survived another winter. This is the time of year where spring is in sight but I still need too much gear to stay warm. It exhausts me to dress for outside. But today it's worth it because I'm leaving the house for a lunch date with a new friend, Kristen, who is eager to learn about parenting to decide if she's ready to have a baby. Parenting, babies, that I can talk about. That I am an expert on. After years of unemployment and mental illness, it is wonderful to feel like an expert in something normal.

I have to take the subway downtown to meet Kristen. She works at the Centre for Addiction and Mental Health, CAMH. When she first told me this, it prompted me to reveal that I am bipolar, something I have no problem discussing with anyone who seems interested. We had an easy and stimulating conversation about my mental health and her role as a researcher in a team of psychiatrists. It made for an instant connection.

Kristen sent me the address when we made our lunch plans but I didn't pay attention at the time. I need to figure out where I'm going, so I pull out my phone, find the address, and plug it into the Maps app. As I start to plan my commute, it hits me that I'm about to voluntarily walk into CAMH. A mental hospital. Another mental hospital. Different from the psych ward at the hospital in Alberta, but still. Mental hospital. Mental patients. Mental.

My heart starts to pound. I don't want to see other people who are crazy like me. I don't want to feel sympathetic because I've been through similar experiences. I don't want to relive my experiences because of what I see. I don't want to walk into a new hospital that I might end up in as a patient one day. I don't want any of it. It strikes me that I sometimes hold the judgements I resent from others—like the words "mental" and "crazy", but I can't think about that right now.

I walk back into our living room and sit on the round chair to decide what to do. My back is sweating even though I haven't put on my coat. I try to focus on my breath, but it's difficult after I notice my shaking hands. Okay, I tell myself, you probably won't see anything. You're just meeting her in the lobby so why would you see anything? Good. But what if a patient is brought in while I'm there? Then I'll see something. A vision of a straitjacket crosses my mind, even though to my knowledge I've never been put in a straitjacket. There was one time in the hospital that I felt multiple arms wrap around me and my nurse said, "Yes, I think we need it," and then I felt tremendously restrained. I wondered if they'd strapped me in, but I never asked. I never wanted to know, just in case. I don't even want to know now. Surely no one will come into CAMH wearing a straitjacket while I'm waiting for Kristen in the lobby. Surely not. I'm being ridiculous. Overthinking. I lean forward to stand, to go to my lunch date.

But still, my heart pounds. Because it might be worse than I suspect. Worse than just seeing something that upsets me. What if this is a trick? What if Eric wants to trick me into going to CAMH, to get me inside and have me locked up? Once I'm there no matter what I say, I'll have my file and my track record and maybe my husband against me. Proof of my insanity.

But no, that's really crazy. Why would Eric want to lock me up? Eric LOVES me. He would NEVER do such a thing. He would NEVER do that to the children.

Unless.

I collapse back into the chair.

Unless he's done. Maybe a bipolar wife makes his life too difficult and he's been biding his time. Maybe he wants to find someone more stable to raise the children so they don't turn out like me. Maybe he already has found someone more stable, and he's ready to move on. Maybe this is a trap. Isn't this a common plot line? The woman gets locked in the sanitarium to suit the husband or the family or someone? Didn't I see this in *Call the Midwife*? And *Jane the Virgin*? Didn't something similar happen to JFK's sister and it ended in a lobotomy?

But this is Eric. My husband. The father of my children. The man I've been with for twenty years. The man I told myself to trust above everyone, including myself, when I first spiralled into mania. I am being ridiculous, I know I am. I have to settle down, because now this paranoia is making me wonder if I am going manic again, and that just won't do. I've got to pull myself out of this. I've got to stop thinking.

*Five. See.*

I see the fireplace. Valentine cards decorating the mantel. The piano bench. The grey L-shaped couch. The black and white rug.

*Four. Feel.*

I feel the chair supporting my legs. Floor under my feet. Cushion under my arm. Tension in my upper back.

*Three. Hear.*

I hear the refrigerator. My breath being forced through my nostrils. The furnace pushing hot air through the vents.

*Two. Taste.*

I taste the remnants of coffee. The staleness of my breath.

*One. Smell.*

I smell—. I can't smell anything. Oh well.

I text Kristen and tell her I have to reschedule. I don't think she needs to know that I'm afraid I'll walk into CAMH and never leave, so I tell her that I'm having a panic attack. And then it occurs to me that that's all this is: a panic attack. I've experienced trauma in psych wards and it must be natural to feel triggered. I consider calling Eric for reassurance but I think I'm almost out of the woods. I think I've got this. I want to push further. He'll be there if I need him.

*This too shall pass.* I recall an image of Nandy making chocolate cake in her tiny kitchen, and force myself to breathe deeply. I've got to get out of this house. I grab my coat and purse, and lock the front door after pulling it closed behind me. I drive the familiar route to the grocery store and set about doing a chore I don't enjoy, which for once feels like a relief. The monotony of selecting produce starts to calm me, and by the time I pay the cashier, I am back to my regular self. My regular, bipolar, overthinking self, but still. Calm.

My panic attack, which felt overwhelming an hour ago, is mostly forgotten. I recall the feeling of my heart pounding in my chest and I feel proud. I handled it well. I also feel proud of how far I've come since my first manic episode, from rapping in an ER room with too much confidence, to becoming despondent on our road trip, with no confidence and too much uncertainty about my future. The highs and lows have been extreme. And through them all, I've survived. I've thrived. I've learned so much that has helped me. I want to share it with other people who face similar challenges, and with the people who love them and don't know what to do. I want to share it with the medical community, so they can work on antiquated mindsets and understand how best to help somebody like me. I want to share it with the world.

It starts to rain as I load the groceries into my trunk. The raindrops are hard, halfway between water and ice, and they sting more than soak. People in the parking lot look up and at each other to question what is happening: is it rain, hail, sleet, or snow? The raindrops don't care about the onlookers' confusion. They know what they are and continue on despite judgment and criticism. I smile as I watch the windshield wipers swish back and forth while driving home, pleased by my artistic interpretation of this storm. My panic attack is long-gone, and once again I feel safe. Mother's Day is only a few months away but I'm not scared. I know that storms and sunshine will come and go for the rest of my life, and that's okay. I'll find shelter.

# ACKNOWLEDGEMENTS

My memoir begins in May, 2017, and ends in February, 2020, shortly before COVID-19 changed everything. My mental health was challenged during the initial panic but that's all it was: challenged. I was fine. I was annoyed, frustrated, and irritable, grateful, lucky, and fine. I know many people whose mental health deteriorated and I was proud that mine did not. I worked hard for this, with the help of some wonderful people.

Thank you to my psychiatrists for being so caring, hard-working, and devoted. I feel lucky that Dr. Patel was working that night in the ER and became the doctor to help piece me back together. I feel equally lucky to know Dr. Gordon. I always look forward to our appointments even when I know they will be tough. I do not always look forward to my appointments with my therapist because sometimes they are really hard. But I always appreciate them after the fact. Thank you, Emma!

Thank you to my dear friend Dana Peterson for taking such excellent care of my children during my mania. Also, thanks to you and Cory and your crew at Catalyst Builders Inc., for renovating our home twice during my manic episodes, both times with compassion and perfect, beautiful, results. Thank you to my Calgary friends who cared for our dog, hosted playdates, delivered meals, and supported me more than you realized: Crystal Milne, Selina Kru, Sue Marshall, Shalyn Madigan, Christine Hewitt, Rebecca Baillie, Jennifer Carter-Smith, Shauna Geekie, Shelley Farmer, Jodie Marcyniuk, Michelle McPhee, and Grandma Jean.

Thank you to my Toronto friends: Emma Greensmith, Inez Kim, Marcia Martin Garofalo, Dawn Richards, Bolette Bossen, Kristen Harcourt, and Raymond Hui.

Thank you to my writing coach/editor Shannon Moroney, and our brave, inspiring, writing friends: Jessica Girard and Sima Qadeer. Megan Thomson, thank you for connecting me with Shannon and for your many years of gentle encouragement. Thank you also to reader/expert Joy Norstrom and photographer Mariah Owen.

My parents worked hard to give their children a better life. Mom and Dad, thank you for your many sacrifices. You raised us to be kind, compassionate, and honest. Dad, thank you for helping me learn to trust my logic and have confidence in my abilities. Mom, thank you for teaching me how to be decisive, organized, and strong. Thank you both for dropping everything to support us during each mania and whenever we've needed you through the years. Thank you also to my siblings. Trent, you gave me my first ever writing critique for what was likely a very boring story, and encouraged me to keep at it. Derryn, we grew closer after becoming mothers and then again when my family moved to Calgary, and I deeply appreciate our bond. Kel, we have shared some unforgettable experiences—good and bad—and will share many more. I look forward to the laughter and the cake.

Thank you to my husband for your many years of love and support, and for always encouraging me to write or do whatever I want to do. We are a great yin-yang. I love you. Thank you to my darling children, who somehow bring so much craziness into our house and yet are the reason I stay sane. I love you three to the moon and back.

# ABOUT THE AUTHOR

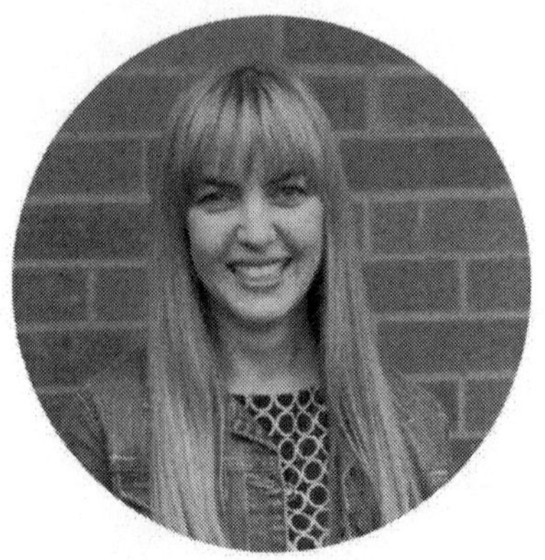

A voracious reader and aspiring writer since childhood, Charise Jewell was born in South Africa and immigrated to Canada when she was seven years old. She holds an Honours B.Eng. in mechanical engineering from McGill University and worked as a robotics engineer for fifteen years before becoming a writer. She proudly lives with bipolar disorder and educates for the fair and dignified treatment of the mentally ill. Charise lives in Toronto with her husband and children. Visit her at charisejewell.com.

## What did you think of

## *Crazy, Memoir of a Mom Gone Mad*?

Scan the QR code or visit
goodreads.com/book/show/58694209-crazy
to leave your rating and review.

To learn more about mental health, mental illness, and resources, visit charisejewell.com.

Manufactured by Amazon.ca
Bolton, ON